The
Beauty Secrets
Handbook

THIS IS A CARLTON BOOK

Published in 2010 by Carlton Books Limited
20 Mortimer Street
London W1T 3JW

10 9 8 7 6 5 4 3 2 1

Text and design © Carlton Books Limited 2010
The text in this book has previously appeared in
1001 Little Beauty Miracles (2006), *1001 Little
Ways to Look Younger* (2007) and *1001 Little
Ways to Spend Less & Look Beautiful* (2009).

A CIP catalogue record for this book is available
from the British Library.

ISBN 978 1 84732 654 6

Senior Executive Editor: Lisa Dyer
Managing Art Director: Lucy Coley
Designer: Anna Pow
Production: Kate Pimm

Printed in China

The Beauty Secrets Handbook

Esme Floyd
& Emma Baxter-Wright

CARLTON
BOOKS

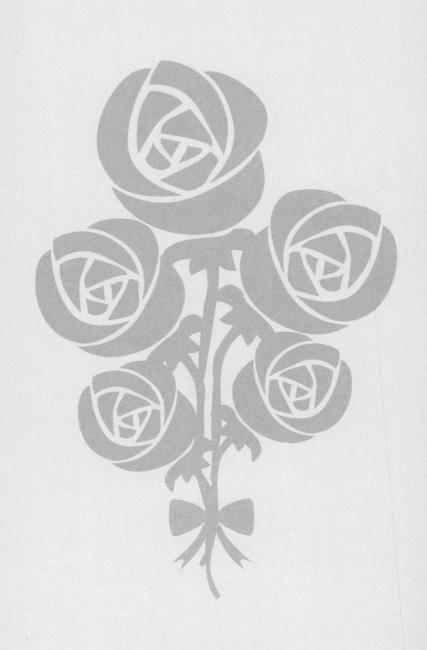

Contents

✳ Introduction

Did you know that ketchup can help correct green tinges in blonde hair, that sun damage makes pores larger or that using a cool, bright lipstick colour will make your teeth look whiter?

Here we've gathered together over 2000 little beauty tricks and tips to hel pyou get gorgeous from heat to toe. Read through the chapters that interest you or dip in and out to get quick, succinct advice for any beatuy concern yu face. From acne outbreaks to untidy eyebrows, from split ends to cellulite, you will find new techniques and solutions to help you put your best face forward every day.

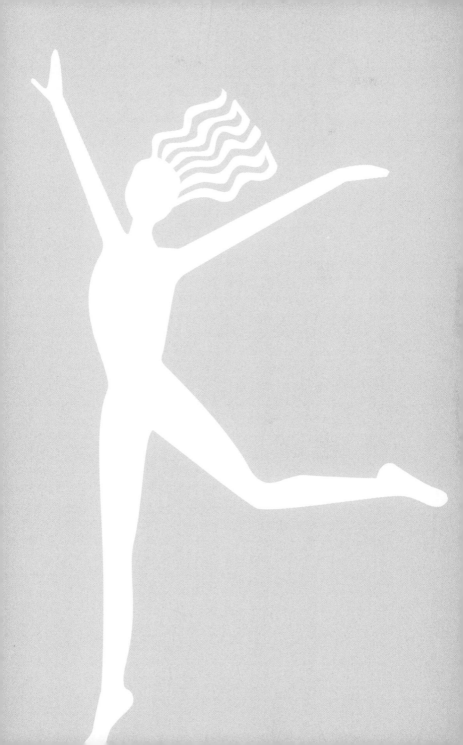

Skincare

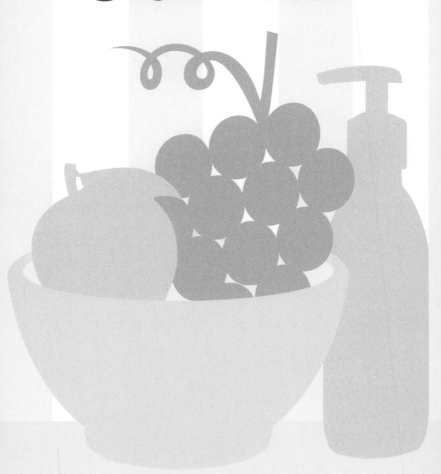

YOUR SKIN IS CONSTANTLY CHANGING according to the environment, season and of course over the years. The following skincare secrets will not only lead you on the path to more beautiful, healthier skin, but will also allow you to understand your skin better. Along with information on cleansing, care and treatments, there is advice on remedying skin problems such as rosacea, acne and eczema, as well as antiageing advice and products to use.

understanding your skin

FIGHT FREE RADICALS

Free radicals, small unstable oxygen molecules, attach to other cells of the body and break them down. The skin protein collagen is particularly susceptible to free radicals, which cause the collagen molecules to break down and re-link up a different way, which in turn makes them become stiff and less mobile. Eating foods rich in antioxidants and using skin products that contain antioxidants can help reduce free radicals.

KEEP HYDRATED

With age, cells stop regenerating at the rate they once did and in the same efficient way. Cells become more abnormally shaped, which makes the texture of the skin appear different and prevents the skin from retaining water. As a result, the skin's texture and water-retaining is diminished. The recommended daily intake of water is 2 litres (75 fl oz) a day for women and 3 litres (100 fl oz) for men.

FAT LOSS MAKES YOU LOOK OLDER

As you age the underlying supportive fat tissues decrease, facial muscles become more slack, and bone deteriorates, so the structure on which the skin sits becomes weaker. Younger people have more fat cells, as do those carrying more weight, which is why many larger older people have fewer wrinkles.

STOP THE CAUSES OF SKIN AGEING

Knowing all the possible causes of premature skin ageing can help you take preventative action. The main culprits are free-radical damage to our cells from exposure to the sun, cigarette smoke, toxins and pollution, but poor diet, excessive alcohol consumption, stress, sleep deprivation, and the use of harsh skin products can all accelerate the skin-ageing process.

SPOT YOUR TYPE OF SKIN

Chronologically aged skin is a result of natural internal factors and manifests as thinner and less elastic skin that is otherwise smooth and unblemished. Photo-aged skin, however, is marked by wrinkles, age spots, uneven pigmentation and a more leathery appearance.

IDENTIFY YOUR SKIN TYPE

In order to choose the right skincare products, you need to know your skin type. Dry skin usually has an uneven skin tone, visible capillaries, and flakiness, while oily skin is more prone to visible pores, breakouts and areas of pigmentation.

SKIN CHANGES

The texture of skin alters frequently depending on environmental factors like pollution and weather so you should change your skin products accordingly. To check up on the current state of your skin, hold a magnifying mirror up close to your cleansed face in bright daylight and look for identifying clues.

SPOIL YOURSELF

As you get older it's important to indulge yourself with regular facials. Women who work hard at being beautiful believe there are no ugly women in the world, just ones that get neglected. If your skin feels great, you feel beautiful all over.

PILLOW PRESSURE

Burying your face in a pillow puts pressure on your skin, which reduces circulation. Over time the wear and tear this causes will break down collagen and cause lines and wrinkles. Switch to silk, satin or a high thread count cotton to minimize the friction on facial skin.

SLEEP AWAY WRINKLES

Keep your neck stretched upwards by sleeping on a high-density contour foam pillow that conforms to your shape and provides maximum support. It will help prevent sleep wrinkles from forming on your face and neck.

KEEP ON DRINKING

Drinking at least six glasses of water a day will to help suppress appetite, metabolize fat, and keep your body and skin fully hydrated and younger-looking. Diet coke, herbal teas and fruit juice will not provide the same benefits to your body as plain water.

STOP SMOKING

Smoking tobacco changes the skin's DNA repair process, leading to the breakdown of collagen and elastin fibres and resulting in premature lines and wrinkles. It also starves the skin of oxygen and essential nutrients, and severely dehydrates it, all of which causes premature ageing.

AVOID SMOKY AREAS

Stay out of places such as bars and clubs where you will be exposed to other people's smoke. Some researchers believe that exposure to cigarette smoke in a confined area is as bad for your skin as the sun's ultraviolet rays. The smoke has a drying effect on the skin's surface, plus it restricts blood vessels, so reducing blood flow and depleting oxygen. Even passive smoking will deplete vitamin C, a key ingredient for keeping skin plump and moist.

BREAK BAD HABITS

Any repetitive movement such as chewing gum, frowning or sucking on a cigarette will lead to the development of fine lines. Over time micro-tears will appear in the skin, resulting in collagen-damaging inflammation. The physical act of smoking causes you to squint and exaggerates wrinkles around the eyes. It also relies on the repetitive action of pursing your lips: every time you suck in, the small wrinkles around your mouth become bigger.

PERFECT SLEEPING POSTURE

Sleeping curled up on your side in the foetal position will create wrinkles and creases on the side of your face where the skin is at its thinnest. Try to sleep on your back at night (and avoid rolling over to dribble into the pillow), if you want to wake up with a smooth and crease-free face.

cleansing & care

BEWARE OF OVERCLEANSING

Overcleansing is a major cause of sensitive skin, as it strips the skin's underlayers of its natural protective properties. Make sure you use a cleanser that's right for your skin type and don't overdo it.

GIVE IT A REST

Moisturizer seals in more than moisture – it stops oil escaping from the skin and can cause spots in those prone to breakouts. Occasionally give yourself a break from night-time creams to allow your skin to breathe and regulate itself normally.

GO LARGE

Remember that for cleansing, moisturizing and facial skincare purposes, your face is the area between your hairline and your collarbone – don't neglect that neck skin. Not only is the skin soft and delicate, it is also very close to underlying structures like the thyroid and voice box. Gentle is best.

STEAM AWAY IMPURITIES

For a quick, deep cleanse, pour boiling water into a bowl with lemon juice and rose petals and hold your face over the bowl, covering your head with a towel. The steam will invigorate you, aid in respiration, and help loosen blackheads. Cleanse afterwards and follow with a cool-water rinse to close pores.

TIP OF THE DAY

When cleansing, many people forget the tip of their nose, which can then become oily or greasy. Use small circular movements to make sure you get your whole nose clean!

SLEEP CLEAN

It's an old adage, but never go to bed with your make-up on. It prevents the skin from shedding and breathing and may cause blemishes and/or blackheads to appear.

SPECIALIZE FOR EYES

For fast removal, use a good eye make-up remover rather than a cleanser. It has oils that dissolve make-up better and faster than regular cleanser or toner. Then wash as usual.

ASSESS TO CLEANSE BEST

Your first step in the morning should be to take a good look in the mirror. Note any dry patches on the cheeks or oiliness in the T-zone. Hormones, seasons, environment and diet can all impact on your skin and will be evident – you can then adjust your regime accordingly.

KEEP YOUR HAIR OFF THE SKIN

Keep hair clean and off the face to avoid making skin greasy, especially overnight when it can rub against skin as you sleep and cause spots and blemishes to appear.

PLEASE WASH YOUR HANDS

Make sure your hands are clean before you touch your face. When applying foundation, use a sponge or brush to give a velvety look.

CLEANSE BEFORE YOU COLOUR

Before applying your make-up in the morning, make sure you thoroughly cleanse your face and apply moisturizer to even out the skin.

CLEANSE ACCORDING TO SKIN TYPE

One thing all dermatologists agree on is that you should use the right products for different skin types. Dry skin should be cleansed without removing the skin's protective film so you need a thick, milky cleanser. Oily skin needs oil-based products as they dissolve sebum effectively. For normal skin, try anything gentle and water-based.

FRESH-FACED GLOW

If you mix a tiny blob of exfoliating cream with your nightly cleanser, you will have a fabulous fresh face that looks smooth and glowing the following morning, with the impurities drawn out.

SHORT SHOWERS

A combination of water that is too hot and washing your face and body with soap will dissolve the skin's natural moisture balance, so keep your daily shower short and water temperature moderate if you want to avoid dry skin.

QUICK AND EASY CLEANSING

There are many facial wipes on the market to help speed up the cleansing process, but make sure you choose the correct one for your skin. Because many are formulated for teenagers, they can be far too harsh for older skin. Even the anti-ageing varieties can be quite chemical and harsh, so it's best to go for wipes designed for sensitive skin.

HANDS OFF

Always resist the urge to poke and prod blackheads and pimples. Even the smallest spot can flare up, and what started as a minor blip on the landscape can turn into a pea-sized crater. Use a small blob of calendula cream for babies overnight to dry it up.

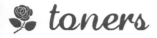 *toners*

AVOID THE TINGLE

In general, products that make your skin tingle are too harsh – tingling in response to toners or cleansers is your skin's way of telling you to go for something weaker. Try toners that are designed for sensitive skin – look for those with a base of rosewater rather than witch hazel or alcohol.

BE ALCOHOL-FREE

Alcohol-based toners and cleansers are the enemy of dry skin, as they strip the skin dry of moisture and can cause problems with skin firmness and blemishes. If you suffer from dry skin, avoid products with alcohol and use a moisturizer more than once a day to keep skin plump and hydrated.

NORMAL WISDOM

If you have normal skin, make sure you choose a light moisturizer, especially one that is formulated as a lotion or gel. Too-rich moisturizers can trigger spots and blemishes by blocking pores.

BE A T-ZONE SMOOTHIE

If you have combination skin, treat the different areas of your face independently – exfoliate the T-zone area, but leave cheeks alone, and when moisturizing concentrate on cheeks and neck, leaving only a light layer on the T-zone.

POUR COLD WATER ON IT

For a quick tone and boost for tired, dull skin, splash your face in cold water to bring fresh blood to the surface, stimulating circulation and giving you a healthy glow.

WITCHES' BREW

If you run out of toner, witch hazel mixed with a little water is a natural alternative, but be careful on older skins which can dry out if the mix is too concentrated.

STOP THE BATH SOAP

Whatever your skin type, avoid using even mild bath soap on the sensitive skin of your face, neck and behind the ears, as this can leave skin feeling tight and drained at best, and can cause redness and rashes to develop. Instead, choose a cleanser that is specially formulated for your face.

DON'T BE A WASHOUT

If you have oily skin, the worst thing you can do is overwash or use a harsh cleanser, as these will actually encourage more production of oils in the skin and could make cause spot and breakouts. Avoid products that strip the skin and opt for lotions rather than heavy creams.

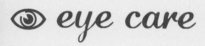 # eye care

HORSE AROUND

For reducing under-eye bags, creams containing vitamin K and horse chestnut are thought to exert beneficial effects by reducing puffiness and blood flow under the thin skin of the area.

GO GENTLY INTO THE NIGHT

When you apply night cream under your eyes, do so gently. Use your fourth finger (which is the weakest) and pat the cream back and forth under the eye, starting at the outer corner and working inwards.

KEEP IT LOW

Don't put eye cream on your upper lids before bedtime or you'll wake up with puffy lids. The cream will prevent the delicate skin in the area from breathing.

SOOTHE EYES WITH CUCUMBER

Place a slice of cucumber on each eyelid for 10–15 minutes to allow the high water and mineral content of the cucumber to be absorbed into your delicate eye skin.

USE AN EXTRA PILLOW

Using an extra pillow can help avoid puffy morning eyes by assisting fluid to drain out of the face by angling it downwards. If your neck gets sore, move the pillow under your chest or shoulders.

STRENGTHEN UNDER-EYE CAPILLARIES

Some under-eye creams, such as Hylexin, contain ingredients that are meant to help strengthen the capillaries that leak blood under the eyes and cause the dark black and blue tints. Make sure the formulas include ingredients that support elastin and collagen too, as these will help firm the skin and improve its ability to "spring back".

WAKE UP EYES WITH AYURVEDA

To keep your peepers perky with an Ayurvedic remedy, sprinkle cold water ten times over tired eyes (keeping them open) morning and night. If you wear contact lenses, do this before you put them in!

ONE-SHOT WONDER

An innovative gel called Laresse is available for small eyebrow creases, and wrinkly crow's-feet. Made in the lab rather than from human or animal sources, it has been praised for its super-smooth results.

HERBAL TREATMENT

Reduce puffy or swollen eyes with a green tea compress. Dip cotton wool into the green tea, drain off excess moisture, then dab gently around the eye area. This will help to tighten the skin around the eyes.

SMOOTH FINE EYE LINES

After a night out in a smoky atmosphere, eyes can become tired and red. Soothe them by grating cucumber onto a muslin cloth. Wrap it up like a tortilla wrap and hold it gently against your eyes. The enzymes in the cucumber will help to reduce swelling and smooth out fine lines.

WAKE UP WITH REFRESHED EYES

Keep a bottle of toning eye make-up remover in the fridge, and use the solution to gently clean your eyes in the morning. The chilled remover will help de-puff the eyes as well as clean.

PAD YOUR EYES

There are several under-eye beauty pads on the market that contain powerful botanicals, such as soybean extracts, to temporarily reduce puffiness and dark circles after a week. They are contoured to the under-eye area. You will need to wear them for 30 minutes a day in order to see results.

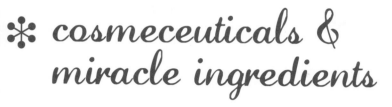

cosmeceuticals & miracle ingredients

GET SMOOTH WITH SOY

Soy proteins can help make skin temporarily smoother by improving
firmness and elasticity if applied regularly. Look for them as
ingredients in new hi-tech face creams.

CUCUMBER AND THYME

Cucumber and thyme contain anti-inflammatory and antiseptic
properties to soothe red, irritated skin, and are thought to be
especially powerful when used in combination with each other,
as they exert stronger effects.

QUEUE UP FOR CO-Q10

Co-enzyme Q10 is a natural antioxidant found in every cell of the
body that helps fight bacteria and free radicals and allows
cells to grow and repair. Incorporated in anti-wrinkle creams,
the synthetic version can reduce lines and deter new ones.

PAPAYA FOR PAPAIN ENZYME

Papaya contains the papain enzyme, a natural, nonabrasive botanical
that dissolves dead skin cells, which makes it a great ingredient for
face masks and exfoliators. It deep cleanses without stripping, leaving
dull skin smoother and more refined.

GO MAD FOR MANGOSTIN

If you suffer from redness, blotchiness and broken capillaries on
the skin, look for Mangostin in your face cream. An extract from
the mangosteen fruit, Mangostin has been shown to help reduce red
patches, dark spots and other circulation-related troubles, particularly
when combined with antioxidant vitamins A, C and E.

COTTON RICH

Cotton is a natural ingredient that has hit the headlines – especially for dry skins. The structure of cottonseed oils can help skin lock away moisture and stay hydrated for longer.

KNOW YOUR NASTIES

If you're worried about chemicals and toxins in products, the main ones to steer clear of on ingredients lists are: propylene glycol (used in antifreeze), isopropyl alcohol, methylisothiazolinone, sodium lauryl sulphate (used in engine degreaser), formaldehyde, stearalkonium chloride, DEA (diethanolanine) and TEA (triethanolinine).

C THE DIFFERENCE

Vitamin C (ascorbic acid) has a brightening effect on skin as it helps boost circulation and collagen production, which means skin looks and feels firmer and smoother as a result. It is essential to the formation of collagen. Vitamin C is found in high levels in citrus fruits, berries and kiwi, but also in serums, creams and other beauty products.

GET HELP FROM AHA

Alpha-hydroxy acids (AHAs), found in many anti-ageing products, are organic chemicals derived from fruit-bearing plants, hence often called "fruit acids". Thought to help generate new collagen, making skin firmer and plumper, they also dissolve the "glue" that binds dead cells, allowing the old ones to be washed or cleansed away and revealing younger cells.

WEAR A MICRO MINERAL

Micronized titanium and zinc oxide mineral make-up provide sun protection and minimize itching and burning. Due to the fact that these powders are composed completely of micronized rock, they cannot grow bacteria, which makes them safe for use on sensitive and healing skin.

LIGHTEN UP WITH LIQUORICE

Liquorice extract has been shown to have an evening and lightening
effect on skin that will help fade age and sun spots if used over a few
months. Many anti-ageing creams now contain it.

TAKE UP TOCOPHEROL

The ingredient alpha-tocopherol, found in face creams and
sunscreens, is thought to optimize protection against damaging UVA
and UVB rays, help prevent premature signs of ageing and stimulate
collagen production to make the skin look younger.

AXE WRINKLES WITH ASTAXANTHIN

Astaxanthin is a carotenoid pigment and powerful "super" antioxidant.
Derived from natural oils, it is thought to have regenerating and
rejuvenating effects on the skin, is an anti-inflammatory, plumps up
skin and reduces the appearance of blemishes and wrinkles. It offers
superb protection against environment damage.

SHARK IT UP

Look for anti-ageing creams with shark cartilage included. The
ingredient stimulates the natural production of collagen and elastin in
the skin, making it look and feel younger, firmer and plumper. It is an
anti-inflammatory and anti-angiogenic.

PLANT PROTEINS

Some plant proteins used in skincare products have been shown
to be almost as effective over short periods as salon treatments
for smoothing skin and reducing wrinkles.

REPAIR TISSUES WITH B5

Vitamin B5 is known to assist with tissue repair, which can help the
skin to feel smoother and younger because it repairs problems in the
deeper layers and prevents blemishes and fine lines.

SILICA SOLUTIONS

Concentrated organic silica builds up keratin in hair and nails by providing the basic building blocks for new keratin to be formed. These products are often derived from sea shells, which also contain other marine boosters.

VITAMIN COCKTAILS

BioVityl and VitaNiacin technology is a good way to give skin a vitamin boost, by combining vitamins the skin needs in one formula. The combination of vitamins cleverly increases absorption and makes the creams work better.

THINK ZINC

Zinc sulphate products like Cellex-C are naturally derived from plants and sometimes shellfish and have been claimed to have anti-ageing effects by smoothing the skin and protecting it from dehydration. It can help clear complexions prone to blemishes and can improve colour, tone and texture.

MEASURE THE MARIGOLDS

Marigold – mainly listed on cosmetics packages as calendula – is an excellent choice for calming sore, swollen skin and contains natural anti-inflammatory properties which make it great for sensitive skins.

ZINC IT UP

When it comes to skin-boosting minerals, zinc is the number one choice as it has a direct effect on the regeneration of skin from the inside out, which can not only help problem and ageing skins but will also give your skin a healthy glow and banish dullness.

SAY YES TO SAFFLOWER

Increasingly, cosmetic companies are waking up to the benefits of safflower oil to create and purify emulsions. The product increases the skin's absorption of oils without making it oily, so is a great choice for anti-ageing creams.

REGENERATE WITH RETINOID

Retinoid is a vitamin A compound, available through pharmacies in the prescription Retin-A and in cosmeceuticals as retinol, which can help reduce fine lines and wrinkles by regenerating skin in the lower layers, sloughing off the upper layers and by stimulating collagen and elastin.

SAY HELLO TO HYALAURONIC ACID

Hyalauronic acid is a powerful ingredient that occurs naturally within our cells and contributes to the structural support of the skin if it soaks into the lower layers. Best used as a face mask or leave-on cream.

REDUCE REDNESS WITH BHAS

BHAs, beta-hydroxy acids that include salicylic acid, help shed excess skin cells with their chemical sloughing effect and they are also anti-inflammatories, which make skin appear less red and inflamed, and reduce puffiness. Gentler than AHAs, they can also treat acne.

HYDROQUINONE FOR HYPERPIGMENTATION

Hydroquinone is a chemical ingredient in skin creams (and can appear under a wide range of brand names), which eases the appearance of patchy skin caused by hyperpigmentation. It is often delivered in a hyaluronic acid base to smooth the texture of skin further.

FADE AWAY FRECKLES

Kojic acid and arbutin are natural alternatives to hydroquinone (see above), which work synergistically to help break up hyperpigmentation in the skin's layers by levelling out melanin levels. They have been used successfully for fading age spots, freckles and sun spots.

MAKE MINE A MAGNESIUM

Magnesium has been shown to reduce the appearance of fine lines and wrinkles in skin by helping to tighten the surface of the skin and boost the production of new skin cells. It is often found as an ingredient in age-defying polishers.

LOOK YOUNGER WITH MESOTHERAPY

Mesotherapy, in which vitamins, minerals and antioxidants are injected into the middle layer of the skin, is said to improve skin quality and vitality by replenishing the skin with essential vitamins that occur naturally within the cells. The vitamins A, E, C, D and B create firmness, clarity and smoothness in the skin.

LOOK FOR PRO-PEPTIDES

Long known for their effectiveness in treating damaged skin, peptides are now thought to help reduce fine lines and wrinkles. They can help stimulate the production of collagen and hyaluronic acid in the skin's upper layers, which is vital in the support structure of the skin which breaks down as we age.

LOOK FOR LIPOLIC

Alpha-lipolic acid (not to be confused with alpha-hydroxy acid) is nature's most powerful anti-inflammatory and antioxidant treatment, which is many times more powerful than vitamins alone for skin healing and hydration.

LATCH ONTO LACTIC ACID

Lactic acid is a wonderful ingredient for extra moisturization because it helps the skin hold onto the moisture that's being added through creams and lotions. It's especially useful in anti-wrinkle and anti-ageing products.

GIVE SKIN A FEAST

Skin is the last organ to get the benefits of the good things you eat, so often there's precious little nourishment left, even if your diet is fantastic. Choose face treatments high in essential minerals such as calcium, magnesium and zinc to give it a boost.

ANTI-STRETCH STRIVECTIN

StriVectin is a formulation in face and body creams, which includes skin-firming agents, elasticizers and skin hydrators, that has been shown to lead to visible stretchmark and wrinkle reduction.

BOOST OILS NATURALLY

Major skin health-boosting ingredients in creams and lotions, essential fatty acids, can plump the skin and help stop it drying out with their non-greasy, oil-producing texture.

HANDS OFF OILY SKIN

Touching, stroking and facial massage stimulate the skin's oil glands to produce more sebum, which is the last thing oily skin needs. So, if you want to dry it out, keep your hands off your face.

WONDER VITAMIN

When skin begins to look dull and lifeless, vitamin A can help. Found in retinol, retinoin, tazarotene and palimate, it increases skin elasticity and dermal thickening, and reverses photo-ageing.

SEARCH OUT "ACTIVE" INGREDIENTS

By law the first ingredient listed on a label should have the highest concentration in the formula. The term 'active' means an ingredient that works beneath the skin's surface to produce visible changes. For it to work, however, it has to be protected from air and light, and used regularly.

SKIN-SAVING ANTIOXIDANT E

Vitamin E is known to be one of the most powerful antioxidants, which can help prevent free radical damage caused by environmental factors like the sun. It is found in more and more skin creams to help ward off this damage, but you can source it nutritionally from leafy green vegetables and olive oil.

CHOOSE KIWI FOR THE SKIN

As well as vitamins C and E, potassium and magnesium, kiwi fruit contains high concentrations of alpha-linolenic acid which helps retain moisture in the skin and hair. Kiwi seed oil contains more than 60% of ALAs, making it ideal for skin products.

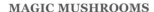

MAGIC MUSHROOMS

Fermented extract of the Kombucha mushroom is a facial treatment that promises to multiply the production of collagen in skin cells, which in turn will plump up the skin and improve its appearance.

TRY TAZAROTINE

Although only available on prescription at the moment, British scientists think tazarotine and tretinoin (whose active ingredient is related to vitamin A) can effectively reduce visible wrinkles, especially those caused by sun damage.

SOMETHING FISHY

Skincare products containing DMAE (dimethylaminoethanol) show good results in the reduction of fine lines and wrinkles. Source it naturally by eating more fish, such as anchovies and sardines which contain high concentrations.

SOOTHE IT WITH OILS

Lavender is the most versatile essential oil, good for helping general fatigue and tension as well as easing skin irritations. Neroli oil distilled from the leaves of the bitter orange tree can help balance both oily and dry skin, and sandalwood is a wonderfully balancing oil which can also help soothe skin irritations.

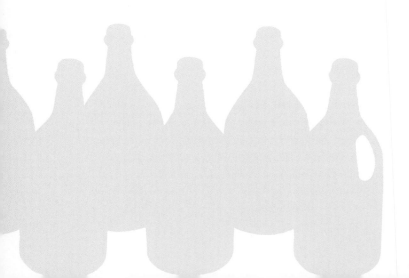

creams, serums & moisturizers

EXTREME CREAMS

Hydroquinone is a common ingredient in skin-bleaching creams, but as it works by killing off the top layers of skin cells, some people find it makes their skin look older and causes sensitivity. Use with care.

USE LESS THAN YOU THINK

Don't slather on more product in the belief that it will work better. Many good products are highly concentrated and only designed to be used in very small amounts.

DAY AND NIGHT

Always use separate day and night creams. The day creams are designed to absorb into the skin quickly and not interfere with make-up application whereas night creams are richer and more emollient and designed for bare skin.

GLOW WITH SERUM

Unlike moisturizers, serums – either in bottle form or as ampoules – have an oily rather than absorbent texture and impart a glow to the skin that improves the visual appearance. They can be used as a quick pick-me-up to give an instant richness to skin's texture.

PROTECT WITH UV

Always use a moisturizer with an SPF of at least 15 to protect from sun damage. With modern formulations there is no need to apply both a sunscreen and a moisturizer.

MOISTURIZE ONE AT A TIME

It's a common mistake to buy three or four similar products, open them all and alternate using them. But if you do this, the chances are that you won't use them all before their use-by date and they'll end up going off or being ineffective.

NIGHT-TIME BEAUTY

Beauty sleep is not a myth. While you sleep, your skin regenerates itself, which is why night creams are such a good idea for moisture. Make sure you go to bed hydrated so the skin gets a chance to heal itself.

FIRM AND MOISTURIZE

For very dry or mature skin, a firming serum or treatment applied underneath a moisturizer gives an added boost.

TREAT COMBINED AREAS

A one-product moisturizer that contains AHAs should treat and normalize both dry and oily areas equally. There are also cleansers available with ingredients that leave dry areas moisturized and oily areas cleared of sebum.

DO IT DAILY WITH LIGHT MOISTURIZING

Every skin type needs a daily moisturizer, so know the one suitable for you. Lightweight gels and simple moisturizers are good for young and sensitive skins.

SERUMS ARE SERIOUSLY GOOD

Serums are pumps or vials of potent anti-ageing agents such as antioxidants and AHAs. Some are formulated for daily use under a moisturizer while others are for short-term or overnight use.

WATER WORKS WONDERS

Kickstart the active ingredients in all skincare products by applying them to skin that is a little damp. Run wet hands over your face or body before putting on wrinkle creams or cellulite serums, and not only will they start working immediately but they will also penetrate the outer layer of skin more easily.

NIGHT-TIME TREATS

Choose products especially for overnight use – these are packed
with vitamins and usually have a specific delivery system that
enables the skin to maximize the extra regeneration of cells that
occurs during the night.

DO IT SENSITIVELY

If you have easily reactive or sensitive skin, stick to simple, pure
products without a cocktail of anti-ageing or AHA ingredients. These
will simply replenish the natural moisture without triggering a problem.

USE IT OR LOSE IT

When putting on a face cream, scrub or mask, instead of wiping or
washing off what's left, use it up on the backs of hands and fingers
to keep them looking younger and well-conditioned for longer.

AVOID REACTIVE SKIN

Use a cream with a mild hydrocortisone included for problem skin
that is prone to rashes and redness. The anti-inflammatory products
will help your skin maintain a healthy profile.

REPLACE OLD PRODUCTS

Skin creams with active ingredients have a shelf life so don't expect
them to last forever. Once a month sweep all free samples and airport
purchases off your shelves, and decide to invest only in products that
are targeted at your age and skin stage.

PRODUCT PLACEMENT

Be careful about laying one product on top of another and overloading
your skin. Too many different ingredients and too much actual
"lotion" can result in irritation and over-sensitized skin.

LOOKING FOR RADIANT SKIN

Facial brighteners are anti-ageing products that target cells in the epidermis that have become hardened and lost their ability to reflect pink tones of light. Brighteners amplify full-scale reflectivity and bring a fresh luminescence to the skin.

NIGHT REPAIR WORK

The skin repairs itself most effectively between the hours of 1 am and 3 am, so products aimed at addressing blemishes and eruptions will be more effective overnight. Use an acid-based night-time skincare product after cleansing to exfoliate the outer layers of skin and hydrate the deeper layers.

BUMPY SKIN

Overloading products can lead to congested pores and tiny rough bumps all over your skin. To keep skin hydrated and smooth, reduce the number of lotions and creams you are using, and instead use a resurfacing treatment once a week, along with a good-quality SPF daily moisturizer.

BREATHE DEEP

Make your replenishing night cream more effective by taking five deep breaths to boost levels of oxygen to the skin before smoothing on your cream.

MOISTURIZE BEFORE MAKE-UP

Apply moisturizer before you put on your make-up because it will give the skin a healthy, plumped-up look. Wait 5–10 minutes and then apply your make-up over the moisturizer.

SERUM COMES FIRST

A serum that contains "active" ingredients for a specific purpose is usually applied to the skin before a moisturizer. As these products are very intensive, only a few tiny drops are needed, so it is worth investing in the best you can afford. As skin ages and produces less sebum it needs daily moisturizing, so you can use both products for a combined result.

SOFTEN STRETCHMARKS AND WRINKLES

Marketed as a miracle cream version of Botox that relies on peptid technology (which helps photo-aged skin and is claimed to perform better than vitamin C or retinol), Strivectin was originally used to improve the appearance of stretchmarks. Although no cream can relax wrinkles away, there is some evidence that Strivectin may help prevent new lines forming and reduce the deepness of existing wrinkles.

FIGHT CITY POLLUTION

Urban pollution plays havoc with your skin. Windborne dust, particles of dirt and smog can all clog up your pores and make your skin choke. Use a daily moisturizer that is specially formulated for city skin to act as a barrier against pollution. Don't forget to cleanse thoroughly at the end of the day.

FIRM UP WISELY

Firming face creams are ideal for skin that is saggy and has lost its natural elasticity as the cream temporarily tightens as well as moisturizes. They usually contain hyaluronic acid to help rebuild collagen and create a firmer foundation.

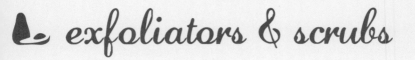 # exfoliators & scrubs

BE AVOCADO FAIR

For a natural exfoliant, grate an avocado stone with a small grater and add it to a little yogurt, cream or avocado flesh. Use the mixture to polish the skin, then rinse off.

EXFOLIATE FOR EXCEPTIONAL SKIN

If left on the body, dead skin cells flake, dry and peel quickly, so the best way to keep skin looking smooth, vital and evenly coloured is to scrub away those dead cells with a shower scrub.

MAKE YOUR OWN

For a super-smoothing skin exfoliant, massage a handful of Epsom salts with a tablespoon of olive oil over wet skin to cleanse, exfoliate and soften the rough spots. Rinse off well for a polished finish.

GIVE NATURE A HAND

Every 24 hours, we lose an astounding 10 billion cells from the skin's surface, though as we age our skin cells take longer to renew. Exfoliating once a week or more helps boost this natural process, preventing blemishes and dull skin caused by the build-up of dead skin cells and revealing a clearer complexion.

SHIELD IN THE SUN

Newly exfoliated skin is more prone to sun damage, so apply a sun block after exfoliating if you're going to be exposed.

STOP INGROWERS

Regular exfoliation has been shown to help prevent ingrown hairs and promote smoother skin as the skin "gets used" to regenerating itself in response to the upper layers being removed efficiently.

BRUSH AND GO

If your lips are seriously dry or flaky, apply a little lip balm and brush them with a soft, dry toothbrush to boost circulation and remove all the dead skin cells while working the moisturizer into the deeper levels of your skin.

TINGLE AWAY

Generally, tingling after exfoliation means you've used too harsh a product, but it is natural to tingle for up to 15 minutes after using alpha- or beta-hydroxy acids to exfoliate because of their chemical effect; the tingling is generally a sensory irritation.

EXFOLIATE WITH CARE

Don't be tempted to rub too hard or use a too-grainy exfoliant on your face. Instead, choose small-grained products and keep it to once a week. If your skin looks red or patchy, you've gone too far.

FACE FACTS WEEKLY

On your face, you should exfoliate once a week to remove dead skin cells. This will not only make your skin look fresher and more radiant, but also helps your products penetrate deeper into the epidermis, making them more effective.

DON'T MIX FACE AND BODY

Don't be tempted to use body exfoliators on facial skin, because products designed for the body are likely to be harsher and could be too abrasive for your face, resulting in irritation.

EXFOLIATE BUMPS

It's not just your face that needs exfoliating – skin bumps on legs can occur as a result of ingrown hairs. To avoid them, exfoliate legs regularly with a grainy scrub in the shower, then apply moisturizer.

DON'T FORGET BUTTOCKS

It might not be the first thing people see about you, but don't neglect the skin of your buttocks, which can be prone to pimples and cellulite if left untended. Use a bath mitt or puff to gently exfoliate in the bath or shower.

MOISTURIZE ALL THE WAY

If you exfoliate regularly, you should always use moisturizer on your face because the regular exfoliation could lead to skin drying up more easily as a result of having fewer layers. You should use it even on the days you're not exfoliating for best results.

GO GENTLY

Overly vigorous exfoliating can break the tiny blood vessels under your skin, causing thread veins and redness to appear, especially on the delicate skin around the cheeks, eyes and neck. Be gentle and avoid exfoliators with natural grains, as these are more abrasive than synthetics.

BRIGHT AND BEAUTIFUL

Over-the-counter purifying peels can have excellent results. A two-step kit will start with an exfoliating antibacterial wash that contains tiny particles of pumice stone to slough off the skin. The peel solution is then left on overnight and washed off in the morning for visibly brighter skin.

POLISH YOUR OWN SKIN

Exfoliants and microdermabrasion treatments will slough away layers of dead skin cells to leave fresh, unblemished skin that is glowing with vitality. Gentle exfoliation will help to erase fine lines and wrinkles and it stimulates oil production and circulation, which in turn encourages new skin cells to grow.

VOTE VOLCANIC

Some exfoliating cleansers contain as much as 25% ground volcanic rock. These are good for oily skin because they dry up oil without stripping too much out of the skin and causing a rebound effect.

DIY DAMAGE

Always treat your skin gently, as the older you are the thinner it gets. Vigorous rubbing during exfoliation or microdermabrasion treatments will increase the skin's sensitivity, and lead to a loss of pigmentation.

REFINE WITH A PORE MINIMIZER

Specially formulated cleansers to reduce the appearance of large pores usually do so via a thermal warming agent, which opens the pores. The cream has in-built cleansers and exfoliators that clean and slough away the debris and tighten the skin, for a more refined appearance.

NEW CELLS, NEW SKIN

Young skin renews itself every month. As we get older the process slows down, so gentle exfoliation will help to maintain the cycle of renewal, scrubbing away dead cells and leaving you with smooth skin – but for older skin keep the treatment to once a week.

NATURAL VERSUS SYNTHETIC

Natural abrasive scrubs like walnut kernels work best on younger skins. Synthetic options commonly found in microdermabrasion creams contain particles that are smooth and spherical. Especially designed for older skin, they will not cut or scratch it.

SEARCH OUT SALICYLIC ACID

This is the only betahydroxy acid that works mainly as an exfoliant to improve the skin's colour and texture. It is an oil-soluble acid that can penetrate into the pores which contain sebum, and exfoliate the dead skin cells that build up inside.

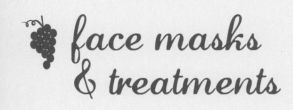

face masks & treatments

EGGS-ELEVEN
Eggs make masks to suit all skin types. An egg white whipped and patted on the skin will tighten and tone. The whole egg, beaten, has softening properties as well. Add egg to any mask for an "eggstra" treat!

MASKS ARE ANTI-AGEING
For mature skin, masks can deliver a burst of temporary anti-ageing ingredients that instantly soften and smooth lines. Often the firming effects can last for several days.

GO EASY FOR SENSITIVE SKIN
If you find your skin reacts badly to mask, but you still want to use them, try those with gentler ingredients like camomile and cucumber, and avoid lanolin, which can often cause reactions.

BE A SMOOTH-SKINNED HONEY
Honey and almond flour, mixed together into a paste, makes an excellent scrub for oily skin because of honey's antiseptic properties and the high levels of vitamins they both contain. Its graininess makes it an excellent gentle exfoliator.

POST-MASK MOISTURE BOOST
Always moisturize directly after using a mask, unless the mask is a leave-on product and you are instructed to rub in the residue. With dead skin cells sloughed off and pores unclogged, your moisturizer will sink in more deeply and have greater penetrating results.

CLEANSE BEFORE YOU COVER
You wouldn't polish a dirty floor and neither should you put a mask on a dirty face. You'll only get the full benefits if you apply the mask to cleansed skin, which will allow your face to absorb more of the ingredients in the mask.

FINISH WELL

If you didn't exfoliate before a mask, finish by removing the mask using a warm, wet face cloth in gentle circular movements. This will act as a gentle exfoliant and leave skin instantly brighter and clearer-looking. However, do not use a scrub or product exfoliator at this stage as you do not want to strip the skin.

BOSH BLACKHEADS

For a homemade way to banish blackheads, combine equal amounts of baking soda and water in your hands to form a paste, then rub the mixture gently into skin, on the affected areas only, for two to three minutes. Finish by rinsing off with warm water.

MUD, GLORIOUS MUD

Oily skin responds well to clay- or mud-based masks, but never use them on dry skin as they are too harsh. When the mask is removed, surface dirt, oil and dead skin cells adhere to the clay and are rinsed away with the mask. If you suffer from an oily T-zone but dry cheeks, apply the mud mask only in the T-zone area and use a gentle moisturizing mask for the cheeks.

WATERMELON CLEANSING

Make yourself a cleansing and clarifying face mask using watermelon, which clears the skin of blemishes and leaves it feeling fresh and clear. Apply the pure juice to your face, leave it on for 15 minutes and then splash with cold water to remove it.

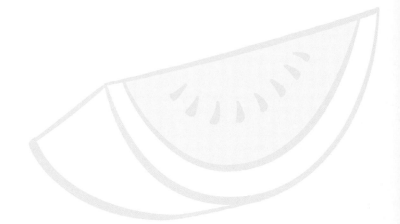

BANANAS FOR SMOOTH SKIN

Banana is one of the best ingredients for an anti-wrinkle treatment because of its vitamins, minerals and smooth, soothing consistency. Mash down two or three slices with a little milk. Apply all over your face and leave for 15–20 minutes before rinsing off with warm water.

MIX UP A VITAMIN BLEND

Create a replenishing face mask with the flesh of one avocado, a little orange juice, honey, molasses and a few drops of camomile essential oil whizzed together in a blender to give your skin a vitamin boost.

TISSUES FOR DRY ISSUES

Masks for dry skin can be tissued off if your skin is extra-dry, so a thin film of the moisture stays behind quenching skin for hours afterwards. Be careful not to leave too much product on as it can clog pores.

BREW UP A STORM

For oily skin, a brewer's yeast mask can help tone without drying out. Mix a teaspoon of brewer's yeast with enough natural yogurt to make a loose, thin mixture. Pat this thoroughly into the oily areas and allow it to dry on the skin. After 15–20 minutes, rinse off with warm water, then cool and blot dry.

GO GENTLY WITH CUCUMBER

For gentle rehydration for sensitive skins, combine half a cucumber, scooped out of its skin, one tablespoon of yogurt, a few strawberries, and one teaspoon of honey. Apply to your face and allow to dry, then gently wipe off.

THE DO-NOTHING FACELIFT

Retrain your face muscles to assume their correct, relaxed and natural appearance with stick-on "Frownies". Designed to be worn overnight on the forehead and between the brows, they work to smooth underlying facial muscles and so reduce expression lines, leaving younger-looking skin.

GIVE YOURSELF A GRAPE BOOST

Forget expensive lotions – grape juice makes an excellent cleanser for any skin type. Simply split one or two large grapes, remove their pips and rub the flesh over your face and neck for an instant, antioxidant cleanser. Rinse off with cool water.

HIT BLEMISHES WITH A CARROT STICK

A carrot mask can work wonders for blemished complexions. Use a small raw carrot mashed to a smooth paste or boil one in a little water and mash it. Then pat the mask all over the blemished areas and leave on for 15–20 minutes. Rinse and pat dry.

DO A PATCH TEST

People with sensitive skin should take care when using masks. Test a small amount of the mask on the area behind your ear and watch for 24 hours to see if there's a reaction. Always remove masks immediately if you feel tingling or burning.

LAY IT ON THICK

Masks work best when coverage is generous, so don't be afraid to use a thicker application. This is one case when trying to skimp is a false economy because the mask won't do as much for the skin if it's thin and you'll only be more tempted to use it more often.

PACK IT WITH PETALS

Prepare a rose face mask by grinding a handful of petals into a paste with a little milk and, if desired, a teaspoon of honey. Apply to clean skin and leave for 15–25 minutes. Wash the paste off with plain water (no soap) and your complexion will be smooth, soft and glowing.

ZAP NEW FREE RADICALS

Studies show that mobile phones and computers emit electromagnetic waves that can penetrate the skin. Protect your skin with Clarins Expertise 3P, a skin-fortifying mist with plant extracts that helps the cell walls stay intact.

COLD SPOON COMPRESS

For a quick fix for puffy eyes, keep two metal teaspoons in the fridge. Place the metal on the swollen area and gently press for at least 60 seconds to reduce puffiness.

MAGNETIC FACELIFT

Promising to smooth out wrinkles and deliver a boost to ageing skin, a magnetic face mask consists of 19 strategically placed magnets which need to be worn for between 30 and 60 minutes a day for at least a couple of weeks to see an improvement.

STIMULATE COLLAGEN PRODUCTION

Facial acupuncture is thought to give you clearer, brighter skin, and to stimulate collagen fibres resulting in increased elasticity of skin, as well as plumping out wrinkles.

NEVER EXPERIMENT ON THE DAY

Face masks, skin bleaching, soothing eye pads or any other beauty procedure that will affect the way your skin looks should not be carried out for the first time immediately prior to a special occasion. Even "normal" skin can turn red and lumpy so only experiment on quiet nights when your social calendar is free.

PRE-PARTY PREP

Prior to a big event choose a "lifting" and lymphatic drainage-based treatment which will improve the appearance of skin tone and reduce puffiness, rather than one that deals with extractions, which is more likely to bring impurities to the surface and may cause your skin to break out – and ruin your evening!

TROPICAL FACE MASK

The common coconut has fantastic benefits for older skin. Cut up the flesh in a blender, then add boiling water and process for 10 minutes; squeeze the resulting mixture through cheesecloth. Coconut helps to prevent free radical formation, and penetrates into the connective tissues to keep them strong and supple.

SWEET AS HONEY

Once a week apply a honey face mask for 30 minutes. It is nourishing for the skin, and will leave your skin soft and supple. Simply apply honey straight from the jar on to skin that has been moistened with warm water. Rinse off with warm water, then splash with cold water to close pores.

30-SECOND SKIN REVIVER

Place a fresh hand towel into steaming hot water (not boiling) and then cover your entire face with it for 30 seconds. Use the flannel to buff the T-zone area, chin, nose and forehead, and then splash freezing cold water all over your face to leave pores tight and tingling.

PLUG IN FOR A FACIAL

Using a micro-current machine, the CACI facial treatment carefully massages the muscles in the face using tiny electric impulses which gently exercise the delicate muscles, leaving skin lifted and tighter.

FRESHEN UP

If skin looks dull and stressed, spritz on chilled rose water to instantly revitalize and freshen up. Follow this with a moisturising rose facial oil massaged into the skin with small circular movements, to boost circulation and promote a healthy glow.

FACIAL ACUPUNCTURE

Tiny needles are inserted all over the face to clear blocked energy in your body and to alleviate stress, which causes wrinkles. Facial acupuncture aims to clear blockages and restore balance so that the body functions efficiently and skin looks healthy and radiant.

SPA TREATMENT AT HOME

This light therapy system stimulates collagen and elastin production and helps to diminish fine lines. The machine has two panels of visible red and infrared lights, which penetrate the skin with pulses of non-thermal light energy, triggering a response from the skin. The treatment takes 10 minutes a day.

AVOCADO PICK-ME-UP

Take a ripe avocado and simply place slices of it onto your skin, particularly on the very dry parts. Older skin becomes drier and more translucent and the oil in the fruit will activate increased oil production within your skin, giving you a softer and younger look.

WAKE UP WITH WATER

To revive tired skin each morning, splash cold water all over your face. It will cause your skin to contract, leaving it fresh and tingly, as well as boosting circulation and making you feeling energized.

A FRESH AIR FACIAL

An oxygen facial targets the face to improve the appearance of the skin using the latest biotechnology. Pure oxygen mist is blasted into the basal layer of the skin to deliver antioxidants, boost circulation and revive a tired and sallow complexion.

KITCHEN SKIN BRIGHTENER

Dull and sallow skin will benefit from equal measurements of lemon juice and milk mixed together and worked gently into a clean face with a soft bristled cosmetic brush. Leave for 5 minutes before rinsing off for brighter, tingly skin.

TWO MINUTE FACELIFT

A simple egg white and lemon juice face mask that you whip up in the kitchen has a tightening effect on the skin, and will leave your skin feeling fresh and glowing.

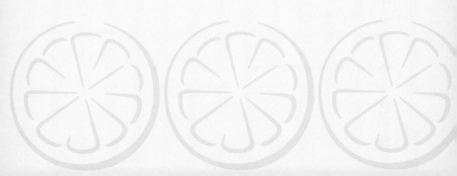

anti-ageing

BE FRANK ABOUT AGEING

Frankincense is thought to have some anti-ageing effects by plumping up the skin and forming a protective barrier against further damage and stress. Find it in specialist creams and salon treatments.

GET AN EARLY START

It's best to start using anti-ageing creams in your thirties and forties to get maximum effects. Before that, their richness will be too heavy for younger skins.

DON'T MAKE THE FACE

Making faces and adopting signature facial expressions creates folds and wrinkles between the brows and eyes. Simply being aware of your facial expressions (particularly in the sun) will stop them appearing in the first place.

SMOOTH AWAY FINE LINES

To prevent ageing and ensure the delicate skin around your eyes stays taut, apply an eye cream above and below the eye area morning and night after the age of 25.

GIVE UP SMOKING

In smokers, skin looks sallow as a result of poor circulation and the action of drawing on the cigarette causes lines to be etched around the mouth. To reduce them, give up smoking if you're still doing it, and avoid smoky environments. The age at which you start to go grey and by how much is largely a matter of genetics, but there are other contributing factors. A 1996 British Medical Journal study reported that smokers are four times more likely to go grey at a young age.

SAFEGUARD SENIOR SKIN

The skin on your face is the thinnest on the body and the older the skin, the thinner and drier it can be. It will need extra protection and moisture, especially in the harsh winter months, so moisturize frequently and avoid harsh toners.

COOK UP A WRINKLE-FREE SKIN

If you want skin as smooth as a tomato, eat them. Tomatoes contain lycopene, a skin-friendly antioxidant that is also thought to reduce cancer risk. Cooking tomatoes makes lycopene more available.

STAY OUT OF THE SUN

Ninety per cent of problems associated with ageing are the result of too much sun exposure, so the best thing you can do to help your skin stay young is avoid the sun.

WRINKLE FIGHT WITH MALACHITE

The exquisite green mineral is thought to be a powerful tool in the anti-ageing battle. The mineral increases cellular water retention, giving the complexion a temporary tighter, firmer appearance.

GET YOUR BEAUTY SLEEP

Sleep is one of the best ways to reduce the signs of ageing, by allowing skin to replenish overnight. If you can't sleep, make sure your room isn't too hot – the deepest sleep occurs if your atmosphere is 18–24°C (64–75°F).

BE ALERT TO BETACAROTENE

Betacarotene, a powerful natural anti-ageing antioxidant, is a pigment in yellow and red fresh foods that the body converts to vitamin A to generate new cells. Get your dose from apricots, peaches, nectarines, sweet potatoes, carrots and leafy greens.

PICK UP PYCNOGENOL

Pycnogenol is an antioxidant found in pine bark that contains vitamins A, C and E as well as its own age-busters. It is claimed to reverse and prevent wrinkles, so look out for it on products' ingredient lists for an anti-ageing boost.

STOP THE SAGGING

The main reason facial muscles sag is a lack of muscular exercise. Regular massage for a few minutes a day is a free and effective preventative. Simply make circular motions with your palm heel evenly around your face.

LOOK GREAT WITH GRAPES

Resveratrol, a polyphenol found in red grapes and an antioxidant and anti-cancer agent, helps mop up the damage caused by sun and pollution exposure, allowing the skin to help heal itself following damage. In addition to eating grapes, look for vinotherapy salon treatments and products that claim to harvest this ingredient.

GET LIPPY

For an anti-ageing make-up effect, keep the eyes bare and wear a strong colour on the lips. This will draw attention away from lines and wrinkles around the eyes and emphasize the shape of lips and lower jaw, giving a more youthful appearance.

KINETIN SKINCARE

Look for skincare products containing the plant growth hormone kinetin (N6-furfuryladenine), which has been shown to have dramatic effects on ageing skin, helping to improve the appearance of fine lines and wrinkles, and reduce blotchiness.

CABBAGE MASK

This mask will counteract wrinkles and dryness and give your skin a healthy bloom thanks to the natural healing chemicals in this leafy veg. Grind two cabbage leaves to extract the juice. Dissolve a pinch of yeast into the liquid and stir in 1 teaspoon of honey. Apply thickly and leave on for 15 minutes before removing.

GO KOJIC FOR AGE SPOTS

Treat skin discolouration, such as freckles and age spots, with Kojic acid, discovered in Japan in 1989 and derived from fungi. It is gentle on the skin and re-balances discoloured skin by penetrating upper skin layers to inhibit uneven pigment formation. Results can be seen after four to six weeks. Vitamin A and mulberry extract are other ingredients that have pigment-levelling properties.

FINGER-TAP MASSAGE

Tapping quickly and lightly all along your facial bone structure helps the lymphatic nodes to drain any congested areas and eliminates toxins. Much cheaper than paying for a facial.

JUST ADD WATER

Applying anti-ageing products to slightly damp skin helps kickstart the products' active ingredients. Not only will they start work straight away, they'll also penetrate the outer layer of the skin more easily so you really get your money's worth.

POMMIE PUNCH

There's no need to buy an expensive anti-ageing skin serum. Pomegranate oil contains a high number of antioxidants and can be found cheaply in most health-food stores. Antioxidants fight ageing by stimulating cell regeneration and minimizing the appearance of wrinkles. Use at night for maximum benefits.

CHECK WHAT'S WORKING

So you're spending a small fortune on several miracle face creams, but do you know what's actually working? Cut back on what you're using and test each product for a few weeks to see which is most effective. Save your money for those.

skin problems

SKIN CHANGES

The texture of skin alters frequently depending on environmental factors like pollution and weather so you should change your skin products accordingly. To check up on the current state of your skin, hold a magnifying mirror up close to your cleansed face in bright daylight and look for identifying clues.

STAY COOL TO CURE CAPILLARIES

For the ultimate in smooth, blemish-free skin, try to stay cool. Overheating can cause damage to fine capillaries in the cheeks and nose, which may contribute to and worsen redness and blotchiness.

AVOID BLEACH FOR VITILIGO

Repigmentation programmes involving steroid creams, UV light and surgery can help address the white patches of vitiligo, but must be administered by a professional. Bleaching agents have side effects and are not the best option for dark skins.

DRIER THAN DUST

For skin tightness, cracking and flaking, choose a cream cleanser rather than a soap-based one and never use drying toners.

HARSH PRODUCTS CAN HARM

If you suffer from rosacea, you should at all times avoid astringents and harsh soaps because not only can they make the symptoms worse, they also dry out skin, making it harder to treat and cover.

TRY SHORT-TERM STEROIDS

Topical steroids can be used on a short-term basis to help reduce the symptoms of rosacea, but long term use may actually make it worse because it thins the skin and can cause other problems.

HELP FOR PSORIASIS

Traditionally treated with coal-tar and emollients, these days creams containing vitamins D3 and A have proved beneficial. Dithranol, derived from the araroba tree, can be used for isolated incidences and has been proven to kill off the rapidly reproducing cells that cause the problem.

EASE ECZEMA

The red, blistering itchy skin of eczema can be treated with a triceram cream, a nonsteroid with a eramide base that helps the skin to repair. Balloon vine extract is an anti-inflammatory that can also help and is available in gel form.

PEEL OFF THE LAYERS

You can now get similar results at home as you would from a medically administered chemical peel because of advances in technology. Over-the-counter "peel" kits contain chemicals such as glycolic acid that dissolve the top layers of skin, lifting them off to reveal a brighter complexion. They usually have a two- or three-part process: the acid solution, an agent to calm the skin and stop the action and a moisturizer.

SENSE YOUR SENSITIVITY

If your skin is reactive, try to find out the triggers, whether they are environmental, nutritional or from using certain skincare products. Bolster your skin's barrier with a moisturizer for sensitive skin and protect it from extremes of weather. Dehydrated skin is more susceptible to infections, immune disorders and sun damage.

KEEP CLEAN TO ARREST ACNE SPREAD

After using brushes or concealer sticks to cover up blemishes or spots, always wash them well to avoid re-infection when you use them again. Or use cotton buds, which are disposable. Also keep your hands away from your face and pay particular attention to habits like rubbing the temples or around the mouth, which you may do subconsciously.

ARREST PREMATURE AGEING

Rescue ageing skin by being scrupulous about using a sunscreen daily, keep out of the sun in summer and rescue early fine lines with intensive serums and brightening AHAs. You must use an SPF15 in combination with acids such as AHA and BHA.

NO ROSÉ FOR ROSACEA

If you suffer rosacea, avoid alcohol as this increases blood flow to the face, which can cause an increase in redness. It also dehydrates, which may make skin appear dryer.

USE LESS ON ECZEMA

When it comes to covering sensitive skin conditions such as eczema, less is definitely more. Use too much powder or base and you risk highlighting the dryness and uneven texture.

FOR SMALL PORES, STAY OUT OF THE SUN

Sun damage – both long-term and short-term – makes pores appear larger because the sun's UV rays break down collagen, making the tissues around your pores weaker and causing the epidermis to thicken. The effects can be permanent.

SPICE ISN'T NICE

Rosacea can be exacerbated by spicy foods containing chilli and mustard as well as hot drinks, which cause an increase in circulation and can make redness worse, as well as causing skin to feel hot and uncomfortable.

STOP ACNE ADVANCEMENT

If you suffer from recurring boils and spots, book an appointment with a private dermatologist immediately – they will be able to prescribe a specific course of action that neither yourself, your pharmacist nor your normal GP has the expertise to diagnose. Allowing the problem to linger means months without a solution.

TREAT SPOTS WITH FACIALS

Regular professionally administered facials can help prevent spots
because they keep your pores cleaner than you can at home. They'll
also help facial muscles relax and keep your skin hydrated and plump.

CLARIFY WITH CLAY

If you suffer from red, inflamed blemishes, use a clay-based mask or
drying lotion to help draw out any impurities and reduce swelling.
Apply only to the affected area if the rest of your skin is dry.

PORES FOR THOUGHT

The best way to keep pores looking smaller and tighter is to keep
them clean, washing your face twice a day – morning and evening –
for best results with a mild cleanser.

PEROXIDE FOR PIMPLES

If you're prone to spotty breakouts, use a benzoyl peroxide solution on
the affected area, which will dry out the area of oil and which also has
antibacterial properties, which can help stop spots appearing.

PIGMENT SKIN ALERT

If you are pregnant or suffer irregular skin pigmentation, avoid
bergamot essential oil as this can cause uneven skin colour to become
worse. Some concentrations are photo-toxic, and can accelerate
pigmentation by making skin more sensitive to sunlight. Avoid
exposure to the sun, sun lamps or tanning booths if using the oil.

HEAT IT UP

If you have to squeeze blackheads, apply a warm-to-hot flannel first
to soften, then wrap a tissue around your fingers and gently squeeze.
Never squeeze facial skin hard enough to leave an imprint.

HIDE BEHIND THE SCREEN

If you notice pigment patches on your cheeks or forehead, wear high-
protection sunscreen at all times to minimize further damage and
ensure your skin stays as even as possible.

WASH WHITEHEADS AWAY

Keep whiteheads at bay on spot-prone skin by washing greasy areas
only with a mild cleanser that contains benzoyl peroxide and glycolic
acids, which in combination have been shown to reduce the severity of
pimples.

PREVENT SPREAD

If you're worried about infection from acne eruptions spreading to
other parts of your face, use a topical antibiotic, which will help to
contain the infection. Never squeeze, as it could make the pore swell
further and look worse, and avoid metal extractor tools which can
damage surrounding tissue.

STAY COOL TO CONTROL ECZEMA

Eczema symptoms can be exacerbated by extremes of temperature and
respond particularly badly to overheating. Make sure you stay cool by
seeking shade and choosing natural fabrics. Changing your laundry
detergent may also help.

UNPLUG BLACKHEADS

One of the most effective ways to rid yourself of blackheads without
damaging or bruising your skin is with pore-cleaning strips, available
over the counter from most pharmacies. Because the skin isn't
squeezed with this technique, it is not at risk from further infection.

STEAM IT AWAY

It's almost impossible to prevent blackheads, but steam can help
minimize them. Once a week, steam your face to soften the oils that
clog the pores and follow with a deep-cleansing clay skin mask, rinsing
thoroughly with warm water to clear the skin.

IT'S HIP TO BE ROSE

For dry skin, choose products containing extract of rosehip.
This ingredient contains high levels of omega-3 and omega-6
oils, which are nourishing for the skin. It also acts as an
anti-inflammatory, which will soothe problem areas.

SCENT SENSITIVITY

Instead of using a scented sunscreen on sensitive skins, opt for an unscented alternative that contains organic, plant-based ingredients, such as aloe vera, jojoba, avocado and camomile.

STEM THE ERUPTION

Cystic acne has the potential to leave deep scars, so spots should never be squeezed. If it's an open pimple, apply an acne-drying gel or lotion and let it run its course. If you have frequent outbreaks, see a dermatologist.

BOTTLE THE MOTTLE

If you have mottled skin or patchy colouring, many heavy, penetrating moisturizers can help disguise and correct uneven pigmentation, giving the complexion a smoother, more even appearance. Opt for one with built-in sunscreen to prevent further problems.

KEEP IT SIMPLE

If you suffer from irregular pigmentation, don't overcomplicate your skincare. Avoid harsh sponges and exfoliating rubs, and don't use toner, which can exacerbate pigment differences.

HOLD THE SCRUB

Beware of over-exfoliating spotty or oily areas of the skin. On problem skin, exfoliation can cause excess oils to be released, making the problem worse, and it can cause acne to spread to uninfected areas. Instead, use gentle polishers to treat the oily areas only.

NO PICKING

Try to avoid picking or touching spots. Not only will grease and grime from your fingers be spread onto your skin, but picking can also cause scarring and pigmentation marks as well as increasing infection risk.

FACIAL HARMONY

To improve red, itchy or allergic skins, visit a salon for a specific ultra-sensitive skin treatment. If plant-based products like arnica and cypress nut are used, they will reduce swelling and redness.

wrinkle-busters

SILK SIREN

For the smoothest facial skin, copy the Egyptian queens and insist on a silk or satin pillow, which will smooth out facial wrinkles while you sleep and ensure you wake up looking your best.

KNOW YOUR WRINKLES

There are four different types of wrinkles – fine, deep, static and dynamic. Fine wrinkles, around the eyes, occur gradually due to the breakdown of collagen and elastin; deeper ones like forehead lines start in the muscles below the surface; dynamic lines are those seen only when your face moves; and static wrinkles are seen all the time.

DON'T CONFUSE WRINKLES WITH DRYNESS

Dry skin can look more wrinkled, but actual wrinkles are not due to dry skin: they are due to damage to the skin's underlayers from ageing, sun exposure and smoking, as well as other pollutants. Moisturize and drink plenty of water to avoid dehydration.

WEIGHT ON FOR A SMOOTH FACE

Rapid weight loss can cause wrinkles by reducing the volume of fat cells that cushion the face. This not only makes you look gaunt, but can cause the skin to sag.

REPAIR YOUR SKIN

Vitamin A can help diminish wrinkle depth, as its light inflammatory action "puffs up" the skin so wrinkles look less deep. Find it in anti-wrinkle creams or add it to your diet by eating lots of fruit and vegetables.

WITCH HAZEL FACE FIRMER

Witch hazel can temporarily tighten the skin and give facial tissues a lift. Instead of using it neat, which can stress delicate skin, mix 1 teaspoon with 100g (3½ oz) of moisturizer and after two weeks you should see results.

WHITE AND GREEN TEA

Green and white tea can help delay collagen ageing and weakening, which has been shown to be a premier cause of wrinkles. Many face creams use green and white tea, not only for their antioxidant properties but also because white tea is shown to limit DNA damage in sun-exposed skin. White tea promotes new cell growth and strengthens the skin.

KEEP YOUR BROWLINE FREE

Squinting is a common cause of wrinkles, as muscles adapt to regular face positions. Wear glasses or contacts to avoid squinting and smooth out your forehead instead of frowning when you're upset or annoyed.

WALK WRINKLES AWAY

Walking delivers oxygen to the complexion, gets blood flowing and reduces tension-related wrinkles because it releases feel-good chemicals in the body, which reduce stress and boost relaxation.

RESIST DAMAGE WITH VITAMIN C

Antioxidant vitamin C in suncreens, moisturizers and capsules will help skin resist damage from sun, pollution and dryness so less wrinkles appear.

GO MARINE

Marine proteins, found in some creams and many supplements, can have skin-strengthening and -boosting properties, which may help reduce fine lines, wrinkles and sun-induced premature ageing.

BE COOL IN SHADES

Sunglasses will stop lines developing around your eyes, caused by squinting against sun or harsh light. Problem areas are in cars and changes in light intensity between inside and outside. Wearing shades in winter, when the sun is lower, is important, too.

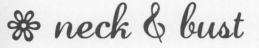
neck & bust

BUST-FIRMING CURRENTS
The Ionithermie bust-firming treatment uses a combination of thermal clay and algae which is spread over the chest. Two types of electric current are then alternated through this layer, to tone and support the muscles around the breast area, visibly lifting the bust.

FERULIC ACID FOR PHOTODAMAGE
The décolletage is very prone to photo-ageing, so protect it with a serum that contains ferulic acid (natural antioxidant most plants produce) – which is particularly beneficial for skin suffering from redness (erythema) or which is photodamaged or hyperpigmented.

UPLIFT WITH FIRMING TREATMENTS
Although there is little you can do to lift a sagging bosom apart from surgery, you can improve the skin texture and tone and temporarily firm the skin by using a serum specially formulated for this area. The skin will look less slack and appear tighter but the effect lasts only as long as you use the serum.

CHOOSE IDEBENONE
Look for skin-firming creams and serums specially formulated for the neck and décolletage areas, especially ones containing idebenone, a potent antioxidant that is claimed to alter the reaction of free radical damage and protect skin lipids. These creams are formulated to re-energize, firm, smooth and brighten the skin.

LOVE BEHIND YOUR EARS
Always remember to use anti-ageing serums and moisturizers behind your ears and the back of your neck, to keep your hidden areas well hydrated and help prevent skin from sagging.

REMEMBER YOUR CLEAVAGE

When applying day or night cream always remember to include your chest area from the top of your bust to your neck. Without extra moisturizer the skin here becomes thin and crêpe-like, and can be a telltale sign of ageing.

MINIMIZE NECK DAMAGE

Don't neglect to nourish your neck with a rich emollient night cream every evening before bedtime. The area from the collarbones up to the jawline often becomes prematurely wrinkled because the skin here is thinner and more vulnerable than that on your face.

 # seasonal skincare

EXTREME WEATHER FLUSH

Travelling between cold exteriors and warm interiors can create a flushed red-faced complexion straining blood vessels in the skin, which change size rapidly as the temperature fluctuates. Find a cream that contains peptides to help plump up skin so the broken veins don't show.

PERK UP WINTER SKIN

In extreme weather conditions cell renewal slows down, resulting in the skin thickening to protect itself and becoming less vibrant. To stop your skin becoming flat and grey use super-hydrating serums packed with hyaluronic acid to nourish and remoisturize.

KEEP OUT OF THE WIND

Strong winds are harmful as they cause moisture to evaporate, leaving skin dry, red and flaky. A skin cream that contains soy will form a protective barrier against the elements and give intense hydration to dry and itchy skin.

TRY A TREATMENT MASK IN WINTER

Winter climates see a decline in the production of lipids (skin oils that seal in moisture). To compensate try a revitalizing mask that contains a high amount of retinol, which stimulates elastin and collagen production, helping to plump up fine lines and even out skin tone in more mature skin.

WISE UP TO WINTER

Harsh weather can lead to broken capillaries in the skin, caused by constant constricting and dilating of the blood vessels as you go from extreme cold outside to central heating inside. To support and strengthen capillary walls, increase your intake of vitamin C or use a serum containing high doses of vitamin C.

WATERPROOF YOUR SKIN

Older skin needs a protective barrier to guard against cold weather and moisture loss. Look for a humectant cream that provides environmental protection, and contains lipids and fatty acids to trap and retain moisture.

TURN OFF THE HEAT

Winter skin suffers from too much time spent indoors in a dry atmosphere. Healthy skin has a water content of between 10% and 20%, and central heating sucks natural moisture out, leaving skin dry and dull-looking. Lower the temperature of your heating, and increase your intake of water.

OVERNIGHT HYDRATION

During the night the skin rests and repairs itself after the stresses of the day. Use a humidifier or place a damp towel over your radiator at night to replace moisture in the air and keep the skin hydrated. This helps to humidify the air around you, and reduces excessive water loss from the skin.

Cosmetics & the Face

YOUR RESOURCE FOR ALL make-up application techniques, this chapter will help you create shapely brows, luscious lips and flawless skin, as well as identify your skin tone and choose colours to complement it. From concealing and highlighting, to cheek colour and eye effects, you will learn the techniques and tools that professional make-up artists use. There is also information on cosmetic surgery procedures such as fillers, peels and laser treatments.

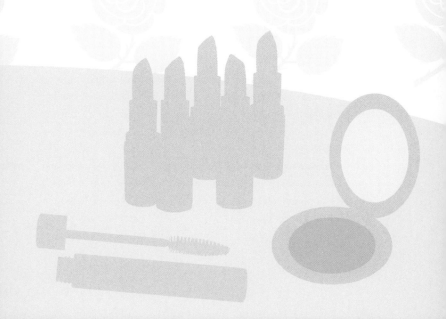

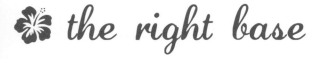 # the right base

PAT IT OFF
After your make-up application, use a soft tissue to gently pat over your face. This will blend the make-up together and soften the look to help you appear natural without leaving you with uncovered patches.

MAKE-UP WITH MINERALS
Because true mineral make-up contains no fillers, it furnishes long-lasting opaque coverage, while feeling weightless. This is a particular advantage for individuals combating rosacea, as well as those who are healing after treatment.

DON'T CREASE UP
Applying eye creams and moisturizers before foundation lessens the probability of creasing because it smoothes out lines in the delicate under-eye area.

DITCH A DOUBLE CHIN
Get rid of your double chin by using a slightly darker shade of powder or foundation under your chin, which will make it appear to recede. Blend towards the back of the jawline to add definition.

DAMP IT UP
For even coverage apply foundation with a slightly damp sponge to spread the base around your face, or use a damp foundation brush for a more artistic approach.

TONE UP
Always choose a foundation that blends with your natural skin tone and never try to counteract your skin colour with a cosmetic. Asian skins have an underlying golden base so you need to choose yellow-based options. Ruddy complexions are best with ivory or pink-based shades.

ADD SOME DEPTH

If you have old loose power that's a shade too light so it's not getting used, add some bronzer or blusher to it. Just add a little at a time and mix to create a bespoke colour that is perfect for your skin tone.

SHADES OF SUMMER

Instead of buying a new foundation in the summer months when your skin is a darker shade, mix your old one with a little bronzer and moisturizer in the palm of your hand and apply to give skin a healthy glow.

FINGERTIP FOUNDATION

There's no need to splash out on special sponges for foundation application. With practice you can achieve a flawless finish using only your fingers. Fingers can reach places that sponges can't and it's also easier to avoid getting foundation in your eyebrows and hairline.

DON'T CAKE IT ON

If your skin's in pretty good condition there's no need to cover your whole face with foundation. Just apply concealer where you need it to hide dark circles or blemishes. As the old saying goes "less is more".

AVOID THE GREY FOR DARK SKINS

Too many foundations for dark and black skins are chalky and ashen. To find the right shade, look for rich colours in a sheer formulation that will allow your natural skin colour to shine through, while evening out pigmentation. Very matt formulas are the worst culprits for a greyish cast.

GO OIL-FREE

In warm, humid weather, skin is prone to producing more oil. Therefore the first port-of-call when summer comes round is an oil-free foundation. Oil-free liquid and sheer formulations are good, choose matt, lightweight options that won't clog pores or leave shine.

BAKE THE CAKE

If your foundation is cakey or too dark, don't just add more and try to rub in. Instead, remove it with a tissue, working from the jaw and hairline outwards with a sweeping motion.

CHOOSE A VERSATILE PRODUCT

Wet-dry foundations are adaptable for all skin types, especially oily and combination skins. They can be used in several ways – sponged on dry for a natural look, sponged on damp for coverage and for building up areas in thin layers, or used dry as a powder throughout the day.

MAKEOVER YOUR MAKE-UP

If your skin darkens more than a shade or two during the summer, invest in a new foundation to match your skin tone. Blend them together for in-between colours, but stick to the same brand so the texture and formula remains the same.

GOODNIGHT, SWEET CREAMS

For maximum coverage, that you might choose for an evening party with low-level lighting, cream foundation is the best option.

MATT FOR MATURE

Matt foundation is good for more mature skins, as it will cover imperfections and control shine without the skin looking too "made-up" or overdone.

DON'T HIDE FROM THE LIGHT

Light-diffusing and -reflecting foundations deflect light away from fine lines and wrinkles, and contain micropigments that give a smooth finish. They have an instant anti-ageing effect and add a subtle glow.

A WHITER SHADE OF PALE

If you prefer a pale, porcelain face with a flawless finish, use a white-coloured skin primer to give an all-over, even base before you apply a foundation. The primer will help avoid the need for touch-ups.

PREPARE YOUR CANVAS

Being heavy-handed with the moisturizer before you apply foundation can lead to streaking. Get the amounts right by applying a light application of moisturizer with a make-up sponge and leave it to dry for at least ten minutes before applying foundation and colour cosmetics.

LIKE LIQUID FOR DAY

For the sort of sheer-to-medium coverage that looks great in the daytime, try liquid foundations. These spread on easily and will last all day without becoming heavy or settling into fine lines. Always shake the bottle gently first to distribute the contents and apply to the centre of the face using light, dabbing movements with the finger-tips before gently blending outwards.

GET PUMP ACTION

If you can, choose a foundation in a tube or pump dispenser. These are good because the product can't slip back into the container after it has been exposed to air or touched, thus reducing the risk of contamination.

LONG FOR LONGLASTING?

A cream-to-powder foundation formula is a good option for dry and mature skins. It goes on as a rich, creamy moisturizer, but dries to a matt velvety finish that looks immaculate and provides good, longlasting coverage, which won't "slip" or rub off during the day like many cream-based foundations.

BRONZE AWAY REDS

If you have a ruddy complexion or uneven, browny-red skin tones, think about using a beige foundation or a bronzer to maintain the natural look while evening out skin tone. Many very pale foundations have a pinky undertone that will exacerbate redness.

NEUTRALIZE YELLOW

Get rid of yellow skin tones, especially in sallow skin around the eyes, using a violet skin correction colour.

GO GREEN TO REDUCE REDNESS

A green-coloured corrector under foundation can reduce cheek redness, but use sparingly and blend well, or you will make yourself look unnaturally pale.

FACE FACTS ABOUT COMPACTS

Those with acne-prone skin should avoid compact foundations because the sponge can provide a breeding ground for bacteria and a heavy base may accentuate pimples and wrinkles. Go sheer instead.

FORGET YOUR LINES

If you have lines on your forehead, apply a light, oil-based foundation and set with a little translucent, light reflective powder to hide the lines away.

CREAMY CHEEKS

If the skin on your cheeks is dry, go for a creamy or oil-based foundation that will help smooth out dry skin and stop make-up flaking and peeling. Moisturize first for best results.

LOOK FRESH AS A DAISY

Freshen foundation at the end of the day by dabbing moisturizer under the eyes and smoothing it across the cheekbones for a touch of added sheen.

OPEN WIDE

When applying foundation, open your mouth to expose the neck area and allow you to blend your base over the jawline, to avoid an obvious line. Alternatively, do it afterwards to check you've blended properly.

BE CLEVER WITH YOUR CLOTHES

Wearing light-coloured clothing helps to reflect light back onto the face, which can lighten dull skin and illuminate make-up.

DON'T HOARD FOUNDATION

Throw foundation away if it starts to look or smell different, or if the ingredients start to separate. It may be out of date, which means it will have lost some of its texture and efficiency and will not glide on well.

BLEND, BLEND, BLEND

After you have applied your foundation, make sure you spend a few minutes blending it onto your jawline, hairline and slightly onto your neck. Spend twice as long on your foundation as you do on any other element of your make-up.

TAKE CARE ON BROKEN SKIN

Be careful when using foundation near broken or infected skin as the infection could spread into the pot. Scoop a small amount onto a plastic dish, then put the container away so you don't accidentally contaminate the pot.

YOUR DUTY TO BE DEWY

After you've applied foundation, to add a dewy glow, moisten a gauze pad or wash-cloth in a mild astringent like witch hazel and gently pat your face. The witch hazel will remove the matt look of your make-up and leave skin covered but radiant.

BEWARE OF FACIAL HAIR

Try to avoid using thick foundations or powder on areas where you have facial hair. These products can cause the hairs to become more visible by forming a coating over them. If coverage is essential, wipe off any excess with a tissue.

DON'T SLEEP IN MAKE-UP

Sleeping in your make-up is the ultimate beauty no-no. You'll end up having to spend loads on products to save your damaged, pimply skin. Keep a pack of face wipes by your bed for nights when you're just too tired to cleanse.

concealing & covering

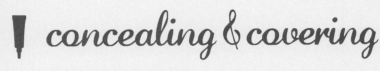

DON'T GO TOO LIGHT

The most common mistake women make when applying concealer is
choosing a colour that is too light. This merely achieves the opposite
effect by actually highlighting the problem, especially if you're using it
to cover under-eye circles.

CONCEAL DARK CIRCLES

Concealer is the most important step in banishing dark circles
and preparing the skin for a perfectly even base. Gently pat a light
reflecting creamy concealer above and below the eye area to disguise
imperfections. Avoid powdery sticks that can pull the skin.

CORRECT RIDGES WITH CONCEALER

If you don't like the hollow of your chin or think your nose ridges are
too prominent, correct them using a few dabs of concealer just as you
would with a spot or blemish. Finish with a little translucent powder.

STICK IT TO LAST

Stick concealer lasts the longest of any type because it's less prone to
drying out or discolouring over time. Liquid-based concealers may
start to separate or go lumpy when they're past their use-by date.

COVER IT UP WITH GOLD

For concealing under-eye circles, which can often appear bluish
in colour, choose a gold-based, warm-toned concealer that will
counteract the blue and help you hide them.

BANISH SPOTS WITH BASE

Give spots, patches of discolouration and blemishes their own
covering of foundation and allow to dry before applying the same
base all over your face. Use the thicker foundation that has settled
around the bottleneck and lid of your bottle to do this, as it is similar
in consistency to a concealer.

COVER YOUR EYES

If you're covering up under-eye circles, don't just put the concealer under the eye, which can give you a "striped" look. Instead, cover the whole eye area and set with a light dusting of powder.

HIDE YOUR NOSE

To slim down a wide nose, use highlighter and blend a soft line down the centre of the nose, then add a contour shade (a darker powder or non-shimmery bronzer) to the outside of the nose and blend together well.

CONCEAL ALL DAY

Apply foundation before camouflaging problem areas with a cream concealer. Finally, dot with translucent powder to hold the concealer in place all day long.

CONCEAL WITH A COTTON BUD

Using a cotton bud or small, pointed concealer brush, apply a dot of thick concealer to the centre of the blemish, then lightly spread it to cover. Brush over with translucent powder.

COVER UP PIMPLES

It's fine to wear make-up if you have pimples, provided that it is not an allergic reaction to that particular brand. The important thing is to remember to cleanse well at the end of the day.

BANISH BAGS

Lack of sleep is the primary cause of dark circles under the eyes. A quick-fix remedy is to apply a light-reflecting foundation in sequin-sized blobs under the eye. Using the index finger blend gently into this very delicate skin.

PEP UP TIRED EYES

For very dark circles or hollow eyes, use a strong concealer and blend it in a little at a time with a concealer brush. Work by "tapping" the concealer into the area rather than rubbing it into the skin.

REDUCE PUFFINESS

If you are plagued with puffy under-eye bags in the morning, use a
botanical-based concealer formulated to cover dark circles and reduce
puffiness at the same time. The formula should cool, firm and lighten
the area all at once.

LITTLE IS BEST

Don't use foundation in an attempt to cover up deep creases and
wrinkles; instead, use a highlighter sparingly to reflect the light and
give your face a youthful glow.

ZAP THOSE ZITS

Blemishes and spots may appear in the run-up to the menopause
because of declining levels of the hormone oestrogen. Disguise
them with a concealer containing salicylic acid to help reduce
redness and blotches.

COVER UP AGE SPOTS

To keep skin an even tone you need to cover up birthmarks, sun
damage and age spots with a combination of foundation and
concealer, using one or two shades blended together.

LOVE YOUR FACE

Learn to love your imperfections, they make you special. Freckles,
nose shape and lip size all give you character and a unique look –
just think how boring it would be if we were all perfect!

TIP ABOUT CAPILLARIES

To cover up broken capillaries or an uneven skin tone, you can either
massage concealer into the skin or paint the area with a brush, then
blend it in with your fingertips.

DISGUISE ROSY RED CHEEKS

If you suffer from rosacea – excessive redness on the cheeks, nose, chin
or forehead – use a green-toned concealer that will disguise the high
colour and that also has an ingredient to improve circulation. If the
condition worsens, you should consult your doctor or a dermatologist.

CONCEAL BUT DON'T CAKE

Hide blemishes and red veins on fair skin with light-diffusing concealers that have peachy or yellow undertones, which are also brilliant at hiding under-eye shadows.

DON'T BE A SCARFACE

Even the most beautiful skin is susceptible to scarring over time, and no one reaches 40 without having some marks on their skin. To cover small scars, use a special dermatological concealer.

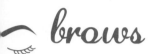 # brows

SHAPELY BROWS

To determine exactly where your brow should begin, imagine a vertical line or hold a make-up pencil straight alongside one nostril. Where the pencil lands by your brow is where it should begin.
To work out where the brow should end, imagine a line from the outside of your nostril to the outer corner of your eye, extending out to your brow.

THREAD IT AWAY

Threading is a form of hair removal. It uses a small thread that is twisted around the eyebrow hairs to pull them out by the root. It is recommended for eyebrow shaping because it's less painful than hot waxes and not as harsh on the delicate skin.

DEFINE WITH A PENCIL

Pencils give the cleanest, most precise definition, but beware of drawing long lines. Instead, use light, feathery strokes to mimic hair growth.

GO TO A PROFESSIONAL

Take the easy route to perfect eyebrows by having your brows shaped by a beautician the first time you try re-shaping. All you then have to do is keep to the lines she's created for you, which takes much less time (and risk).

DIVIDE BY FOUR

For the best shape, think geometrically, as if the brow is divided into four sections along the length of the eye. The first three should head upwards and the outer quarter should slant down.

BRUSH THOSE BROWS

An old toothbrush is excellent for brushing brows after pencilling in. Not only will it smooth down hairs, it will also soften pencil lines, leaving them looking more natural.

KEEP BROWS IN LINE

If you want your eyebrows to stay in place, add a coat of clear mascara or a little hairspray on the eyebrow groomer before brushing to the desired shape.

COMB IT UP

Comb brows upward before plucking or colouring in to make sure you preserve the natural browline. If your brows are very thick or long, trim the hairs that extend above the upper line of the arch.

POWDER IT RIGHT

Eyebrow powder should be one to two shades lighter than your hair colour. A matching colour to your hair can look overpowering on a face and anything much darker is just too severe.

KEEP IT SHARP

Sharpen your eyebrow pencil before every application to make sure you keep the high definition look you're after. You can always blend if lines are too sharp.

CATCH THE HIGHLIGHTS

To make brows appear higher and more defined, apply some highlighting powder or cream under the middle to outer edge of the eyebrow, which will add fullness to the eye area.

GO GREY GRACEFULLY

If you have grey, white, or salt and pepper hair, charcoal or slate grey are good shades to choose for brows, because they will look natural and still give definition.

KEEP TWEEZERS HANDY

Keep tweezers by the mirror for a daily tidy-up, plucking out just a few hairs as and when they appear. This will not only mean you stay looking tidy, but will stop overplucking and help you to keep your eyebrow shape.

JOIN THE BROWNIES

If you have red hair and eyebrows and want to colour them to give more emphasis to your face, beware of going too dark. Choose browns with deep red undertones instead, to blend with your hair.

BROWN IS THE NEW BLACK

For brunettes, apart from those with really dark hair, black can appear too harsh for eyebrows. Instead, choose a dark brown pencil, which will blend in more naturally.

CHOOSE LIGHT BROWN FOR BLONDE

If you have light hair and light skin, select light brown or taupe shades for eyebrows. These will contrast well with your skin without appearing too dark.

GET SHEEN WITH VASELINE

Tame wayward eyebrow hairs with a tiny amount of brow fixative or Vaseline after you've applied your brow colour. This will give them a bit of added shine as well as holding them in place.

POWDER AND PEAK

Powders give a soft effect and need minimal blending. To heighten the arch, apply an extra bit of colour at the highest peak to make it stand out.

PLUCK BEFORE BED

To avoid letting the whole world know you pluck your eyebrows, pluck last thing at night so the redness will have gone by the morning. After a bath or shower, when the skin is moist and the pores are open, is the best time to pluck.

KEEP 'EM HIGH

Never draw brows downward at the ends – this can have the effect of lowering your eyes and making them appear droopy. Instead, aim for a "floating", winged effect to lift the face.

AVOID A CLOSE SHAVE

Never shave your eyebrows – it's hard to control and is likely to drag the skin, causing wrinkles. It also encourages hair to grow back blunt, which can bring attention to re-growth.

MAGNIFY TO BEAUTIFY

To get the best view of your brows, for even plucking, invest in a magnifying mirror and make sure the light falls evenly on both sides of your face to avoid uneven shapes caused by shadowing.

GET BELOW

Always pluck hairs from underneath the brow. Grasp hair as close to the root as possible and pull the hair out towards the temple in quick, firm strokes.

ENHANCE YOUR ARCHES

If you have a natural arch, work with it rather than creating a new one. If you need to create an arch, look into your eyes. The top arch of your eyebrow should fall directly above the outside of your iris for eye-opening results.

GET A PROFESSIONAL SHADE

If you want to permanently darken brows, visit a professional, who will be able to match your shade perfectly for the most flattering results.

COLOURING IN

If you want to reshape your eyebrows, but are worried about making a mistake, fill in the area you want to preserve using an eyebrow pencil and pluck outside the edges. This way you won't over-pluck and you can perfect the shape first.

KEEP IT NATURAL

Never draw a browline above the natural one; it will look false and give you an unnaturally "surprised" look. Instead, work with your natural lines and if necessary use a highlighter underneath to give brows a lift.

NOSE FIRST

When plucking and shaping eyebrows, start at the inner edge and around the bridge of the nose. Form a gentle, tapered round edge rather than a straight one.

TAKE THE TINT

Eyebrows should frame your face and eyes, but they may struggle to do this if they are too pale or have been bleached by the sun. Your brows may also go grey or lighter with age. Instead of filling in with powder, think of visiting a salon for professional brow tint, which will usually last for four to six weeks.

STRETCH TO AVOID STING

Eyebrow tweezing can be painful. To avoid stinging and redness, stretch the skin gently upwards or between the fingers before plucking and pull out the hair quickly to avoid bruising. It is best to tweeze after a hot shower or bath and in the evening, to give your skin time to recover from any redness.

CIRCUMVENT YOUR CYCLE

Pain tolerance seems to be reduced for many just before and during the first few days of menstruation, so it's best to avoid these times if you're planning to re-shape eyebrows. Mid-cycle is the most pain-free time to pluck.

TAKE A BREAK

If overplucking or age has left your brows sparse, first try to resist tweezing them at all for a few months so you can see what you've really got to work with. Sometimes the habit of tweezing is so ingrained that you do it daily without realizing how much you're taking away. You may rediscover the natural beauty of your youthful brows.

REJECT A PERMANENT BROW

Don't be tempted to have brows tattooed on permanently to save time and create a perfect line; the effect is hard and artificial.

FILLING IN OVERPLUCKED BROWS

Bald patches can be filled in by brushing the brows upwards and then filling in the sparse area with shadow powder that's a shade lighter than your natural brow colour. Finish by pencilling over the area with a pencil that matches your brow colour, using short, hairlike strokes.

DON'T LET YOUR BROWS AGE YOU

Brows that are too close together can make you look old and frumpy. The beginning point should align vertically with your inner eye. Never artificially draw in your brow or try to copy a celebrity's brows – the only brow shape that will look good for you is your own natural one.

QUICK BROW LIFTS

Sweep a coloured brow gel over your brows as a last-minute beauty fix. It will tint the browns as well as pulling straggly hairs into place, and tidy brows "open up" small eyes.

SHAPELY EYEBROWS

It's best to combine different techniques to get the best shape possible. Waxing creates the overall shape and a defined outline, but small stray hairs should be plucked and trimmed to ensure a perfectly groomed eyebrow, which will define the shape of the face and open up tired eyes.

THE PERFECT PLUCK FACELIFT

With age, the upper eyelids tend to sag, which is why a perfectly shaped brow can act as an instant facelift. Decide where you want to pluck by shading in the area with a sweep of white eye pencil, freeze the skin with an ice cube, and pluck as close to the root of the hair as possible only within this shaded area.

HELP FOR THIN BROWS

Hair thins on the brows as it does on the head, so if you need to create the illusion of fuller brows, use two colours of brow colour or eyeshadow (never a pencil) – a lighter one for the fullest part and a darker one for the "tails". The shadow will create a full, soft look that isn't possible with a pencil.

COMBAT GREY BROWS

If your eyebrows are losing their colour, never attempt to darken them yourself with an over-the-counter dye as it is all too easy to go too dark. Allow a professional to undertake the challenge and between visits shade your brows in with a matching brow colour in a "wand" applicator like mascara. Because it simply washes off, there's no danger of a long-lasting mistake.

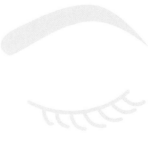

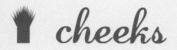 # cheeks

GIVE YOURSELF A SMILE

To make blusher pay, smile into the mirror to find the apples of your cheeks, then brush the colour there in wide, sweeping movements for a natural, cheeky glow.

KEEP TO THE CURVE

Never apply blusher right up to the hairline, which is a sure fire way to make your face look unnaturally painted. Stop on the top curve of your cheekbone.

BLOW AWAY BLUSHES

To apply the perfect amount of blusher or bronzer to cheeks, load up the brush and then tap or blow off the excess. This will ensure you get ample coverage of colour without looking like a painted doll.

DARKEN FOR DEFINITION

To bring out your natural cheekbones, use a medium beige blush underneath to help the bones stand out – avoid dark colours or you will get a stripy look.

JOIN THE MAGIC CIRCLE

Soften the harshness of sharp cheekbones by applying blusher in circular motions on the apples of the cheeks. This will draw attention away from angled bones.

DISGUISE FULL CHEEKS

Use a light application of a slightly darker shade of powder than your foundation on the underside of cheekbones and blend out towards ears to sculpt some definition into round cheeks.

DON'T CLASH LIPS AND CHEEKS

Choose a cheek colour that blends with the colour on your lips or your natural lip colour to avoid clashing and looking "overdone". Or stick to skin tones if you're going bright.

BLOT AND BRONZE

Before applying bronzer, blot your skin with blotting papers or a clean tissue. This will give the skin an even surface and ensure that the bronzer doesn't end up in blotches.

BLUSH FOR TWO YEARS

After two years, powders and powder blushers may start to develop a dry or "slippery" texture. This is caused by too much mixing with natural oils from your skin. If this has happened to yours, it's time to invest in a new one.

DON'T FREAK OVER STREAKS

If your blusher looks streaky or stripy, or if you have over coloured, don't be tempted to add more colour to even out the stripe. The only way to deal with it is to remove some colour with a tissue and dust a little translucent powder over cheeks.

LEAVE THE CREAM TO THE CAT

If your skin is oily, steer clear of cream blushers, which can give cheeks a shiny look and make skin elsewhere on the face appear oilier as a result.

USE GEL TO LOOK WELL

For a natural cheek colour, particularly over sheer tinted moisturizers, use cheek gel instead of powder blusher. Gel gives a healthy, translucent flush to the skin.

GLOW WITHOUT GOING OVERBOARD

When you want to add warmth to the skin, particularly in the daytime, use a light to medium bronzing powder instead of your standard blush.

BE A PEACH BABE

Choose soft natural pinks, beiges and tawny peaches for daytime. These will blend with the tones in natural daylight and avoid making you look overdone. Go brighter and cooler at night for definition.

LEAVE IT TILL LAST

For super-smooth results with no streaking, particularly for evening looks, apply blusher after powder. This will form a smooth, natural base that the colour can cling to.

CREATE CHEEKBONES

Cheekbones are best defined with highlighter rather than blusher, which can cause overcolouring. Blend a line of highlighter along the top edges of your cheekbones and a line of shade under-neath to help them stand to attention.

GET IT RIGHT ON YOUR WRIST

Look for the most natural blush colour you can find. Try it on the inside of your wrist when choosing – if it looks natural here, it will look natural on your cheeks.

THE FUTURE IS NOT ORANGE

When choosing a bronzer, make sure it doesn't appear too orange or frosted. A little shimmer goes a long way; too much can make skin look unnatural and harsh, especially on mature skin.

TWO WILL DO

Never go more than two shades darker than your natural skin tone. Bronzers are meant to warm your skin as if you have a natural glow, rather than adding colour.

GO EASY ON BASE

Too much foundation can leave your bronzer looking "muddy" and artificial, ruining the natural glow effect you are aiming for. If you feel you really need foundation, try a tinted moisturizer or sheer base instead.

HOW TO DO DEWY

Powder bronzers are best for oily complexions. If your skin is dry or you like a dewy finish, choose a cream, stick or gel to achieve your colour.

BLUSH IT UP

For lighter complexions, use a small amount of bronze on your cheeks and forehead. Follow this with a touch of pink or rose blush on the apples of your cheeks, for a natural-looking flush.

FINGER PAINTING

Cream, stick and liquid bronzers should be applied using your fingers. Dab onto the apples of your cheeks and blend, using circular motions, towards the hairline. Leftover colour can be very lightly dabbed onto the bridge of the nose, on the temples and even on the collarbone.

IN THE SPOTLIGHT

If you want to know where to apply highlighter, stand in front of a mirror in bright light to test the best areas. Because you are trying to achieve a natural-looking glow, you should only emphasize those areas that are directly hit by daylight, for example the tops of the cheekbones.

COLOUR ON THE GO

If you're in a rush and need a quick touch up, invest in an all-in-one lip/eye/blush in a crayon, stick or gel to give you a colour lift anytime and anywhere.

PALE AND BEAUTIFUL

If you have very pale colouring stop wasting time with fake tans and bronzers – embrace your paleness and add a fresh-faced shade of blush to the apples of your cheeks where the colour naturally rises.

BRIGHTEN WITH HIGHLIGHTER

Add a little highlighter to brighten up pancake-flat skin, but always look for one with a very fine shimmer rather than garish sparkles which can only ever look good on the very young. Blend over cheekbones and under eyebrows for a look that is glowing but not greasy. You can also mix it in with your usual foundation as a skin brightener.

PLAN STRATEGICALLY
Give your face a cunning boost by dotting small dabs of highlighter in strategic spots – in the inner corners of the eyes, on the lips or on the tip of the nose – for extra shine and definition.

RADIANCE BOOSTING
Products sold as "radiance boosters" or "illuminators" usually have several functions. They can be used as highlighters to emphasis bone structure, as masks to revive lacklustre skin and eliminate fine lines, and under foundation to provide a smooth surface for application, tighten the skin and provide glow.

SUNKISSED
If you don't have time to apply fake tan, using a cream bronzer will give the effect of sun-kissed skin. Use on the cheekbones, temples, down the bridge of the nose, and the centre of the neck for a glowing youthful complexion. Apply with a light touch for a natural look.

THE BEST BLUSHER BRUSH
Always choose a big blusher brush with a flat head and lots of densely packed bristles that is made from 100% natural hair. This type of brush will be kind to your face and not scratch it delicate skin, but more importantly will apply blush and bronzer evenly without ugly stripes.

AN INSTANT GLOW
Skin loses its pigment and colour as we grow older so a quick brush of rosy blusher is most important, particularly in winter when skin is even paler. It will add an instant glow and make you look youthful and vibrant.

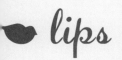 *lips*

PLUMP UP YOUR LIPS

Lip-plumping glosses, with swelling ingredients like cinnamon and menthol, claim to temporarily inflate the pout, mimicking the effects of permanent surgical lip fillers like collagen and hyalauronic acid.

PEAK A POUT

Instead of completely outlining the lips, for a bigger pout just pencil in the cupid's bow, the centre of the bottom lip, and the corners of the mouth with a natural shade. This will enhance the shape of your lips, bringing attention to the edges and giving them a fuller appearance.

KEEP LIPSTICK OFF YOUR TEETH!

Once you've applied your lipstick, put your forefinger in your mouth and then (just like a lollipop) slowly pull it out. All the lipstick that would have ended up on your teeth will have been successfully removed and you will be able to smile with security.

NATURAL OILS

A little olive oil will soothe dry, chapped lips as well as any store-bought balm. Simply dab it on with your finger.

ADDRESS YOUR DRYNESS

Very matt and longwearing lipsticks can be quite dry and lacking in oil. If your lips are prone to dryness, creamy formulas are a lot more flattering and easy to wear.

DON'T RELY ON LIP BALM

Many people find that lip balm is an addictive habit and the more they use one the more they need it to keep lips soft and flake-free. Instead of constantly buying more lip balm, simply apply your normal facial moisturizer to your lips – it will soften them for longer and won't slide off. Make sure it doesn't get into your mouth and don't lick your lips!

AFRAID OF THE DARK

Don't use a lipliner much darker than your lipstick to define your lips.

BRUSH UP YOUR LIP SKILLS

For the ultimate in flawless lipstick application, use a specially designed lip brush – it's the best way to avoid finishing up with too much lipstick. Simply blot with a single ply of tissue after each application and build-up the colour until you get the result you're looking for.

DON'T LICK YOUR LIPS

Don't be tempted to lick dry, cracked or chapped lips, which can be caused by harsh conditions or dehydration, as this will only make them dryer. Take a drink of water and use a lip balm or moisturizer to restore plumpness instead.

DO 3D LIPS

Use your light brown eye pencil to line lips. Apply a bit more on the inside corners of the lip and on both top and bottom to create depth on the outside of the lips and a 3D-effect lip.

GLOSS AND BE GONE

Lip gloss isn't as longlasting as lipstick because it is formulated in a different way and is prone to drying. If it changes scent, texture, or looks or feels different on your lips, it's time for a change.

MAKE DO AND BLEND

If you can't find the right shade, mix it up by using your existing lipsticks to create new colours. Simply blend the colours onto the back of your hand with a lip brush and apply directly to your lips.

POUT IT UP

Create a pretty pout by first applying your lip colour with a lip brush, then using a lip pencil afterwards in a complementary colour. Be sure to follow the natural line of your lips.

CAP IT

Taking care of your lipsticks will make them last longer. To avoid squashing it, make sure your lipstick is rolled all the way down before putting the cap on. Also, make sure the top clicks into place to keep out air and reduce the growth of bacteria.

GET LUSCIOUS LIPS

Just as your face needs regular moisturizing, so too do your lips. Before you go to bed is the perfect time to really allow the moisture to sink in. Before you go to sleep, apply a large dose of your favourite lip balm and wake up in the morning with a perfectly rehydrated pout.

FIGHT FEATHERING

To prevent lipstick from feathering, line your mouth with a lip pencil, which will fill in lines and help to keep colour intact.

MAKE SURE YOU MATCH

Always choose a lipliner that matches your lip colour, then if your lipstick wears off you won't look overdone.

BE A GOOD CHAP

Use a Chapstick as a lip primer under colour. The waxiness smoothes the lip surface, fills tiny lines and will help hold the colour for longer. This is particularly useful under matt colours, which can add to the appearance of dryness.

LIP IT UP

If you're wearing make-up, always apply something to your lips, even if it's just a bit of lipliner and gloss, to make sure you look finished.

TOUCH BASE WITH YOUR LIPSTICK

To form a perfect lipstick base, apply a light covering of foundation with a wet sponge and allow to dry. This will even out underlying skin tone and allow lipstick to stay on for longer.

FINGERTIP TESTER

When choosing a lipstick, never apply the tester directly to your lips. For hygiene reasons the best place to test is your fingertips, where the colour and texture of skin is closest to your lips.

EVEN IT OUT

Even out uneven upper and lower lips by using lipliner only on the thinner one to create the appearance of equality. Alternatively opt for a slightly darker shade on the thinner one to boost visibility.

THINK OF YOUR SKIN

Don't be tempted to match lipstick to clothes instead of skin colour – go for shades that flatter your complexion rather than those that match your outfit for the most flattering results.

STEM BLEEDING WITH POWDER

To avoid your lip colour bleeding, after applying lipstick, dot powder at the upper and lower corners of the mouth, at the outside edge, to fill in lines. Brush away excess powder.

BE A GLOSS LEADER

Create fullness with a spot of gloss in the middle of the mouth, particularly on the upper lips, which will appear fuller as a result.

SAY IT BRIGHT

Lightweight brightening creams can give thin lips a natural-looking pout if blended over the lip line before using lipstick or gloss.

DON'T BE SHY OF BIG LIPS

If your lips are large, don't be shy; promote them as a star feature using a deep coloured, matt lipstick. Avoid gloss and really bright colours, which can overly increase the voluptuous effect.

GOLDEN DELICIOUS

For an instant, glammed-up evening look apply a small amount of gold-coloured or sparkly gloss over your daytime lipstick to get you in the mood.

NICE AND EVEN

Some women naturally have uneven amounts of colour in their lips. To neutralize natural lip colour, dot foundation on your lips and blot before applying colour.

GO THE EXTRA SMILE

Make your lips look fuller by using a pale or frosty lipstick and finish with a splash of gloss in the middle of your mouth to achieve the perfect pout.

SEAL IT WITH AN E

To seal in lipstick instantly, prick a vitamin E capsule and slick it over your lip colour.

STRIVE FOR EQUALITY

If you have a thinner top lip, you can help it stand out more by applying a slick of gloss to the top lip only to accentuate it, then blotting gently onto the lower lip.

GET FLAWLESS COLOUR

To achieve the exact colour of the lipstick on your lips, apply a nude lip pencil to your lips before the lipstick. It will also help keep the lipstick in place for longer and reduce the chances of smudging.

LIP-PUMPING PEPTIDES

Products containing peptides that have been proven to boost collagen production may be your best shot for creating a soft, pillowy pair of lips without a needle in sight.

INSTANT COLOUR

Carry a neutral shade of lip gloss in your pocket. It is easy to apply in a hurry without a mirror using your fingertips, and will add instant colour and shine to dry lips.

FIX THOSE LIPS

Ruby red lips are too bold on an older face and tend to look cheap. If you do want to use a deep shade make sure it doesn't "bleed" into your wrinkle lines by using a transparent lip liner that will seal the colour.

NO MORE ROUGH LIPS

Rough, unkissable lips should be treated with a natural exfoliating rub made from finely ground brown sugar and sesame oil. Scuff this delicious mixture gently over lips to remove dead and flaky skin. Finish with petroleum jelly.

MEND AN UNHAPPY MOUTH

Chapped lips that are dry, cracked and sore will look painful and interfere with many daily activities like eating – and kissing. To remedy the problem, use an oil-based chapstick or one that contains beeswax regularly, and avoid flavoured lip balms as you will be tempted to lick them off and make the problem worse.

RESCUE FLAKY LIPS

Try a two-step lip treatment to treat dry winter lips that are flaky and scaly. A lip exfoliator gently sloughs off dead and dull cells, before an intensive balm is applied to nourish and moisturize the new skin.

LIPS DON'T LIKE LICKING

When lips are exposed to harsh elements we may be tempted to lick them to moisten the surface. This dries them out further because saliva contains enzymes that break down moisture, leaving them dryer and thinner, which can add years to your look. Keep a small tin of shea butter in your bag and use it several times a day in winter.

INCREASE LIP VOLUME

Maximize your lip potential with volume-boosting lip gloss, which will increase lip size and help reduce fine lines and wrinkles that form above the top lip. Lip plumping gloss contains ingredients that react with the skin, resulting in fuller, plumper lips without surgery.

LEAVE OUT THE LIP LINER

If your lip colour has a tendency to bleed upwards and outwards, apply a moisturizing lipstick with your fingers in small controlled daubs with your finger, rather than "dragging" the lipstick along the mouth, which can look sculptured and old fashioned.

LIGHT TRICK LIPS

To give the illusion of a fuller upper lip, dab a tiny touch of pale iridescent sheen in the centre of the lips. This will highlight your cupid's bow making it appear bigger than it is.

DARK LIP DISASTER

Unless you have a perfect pair of lips and the expertise of a professional make-up artist, very dark lips are best avoided. They are ageing and unflattering on most faces as the contrast between lip colour and skin is too dramatic, and the colour often comes off on your teeth.

A LICK OF LIPSTICK

Resolve to find a flattering lipstick to keep with you at all times. Look for one that matches your natural lip colour but with a touch more zing. When you need to leave the house in a hurry, one swipe of this lipstick will give you instant polish.

CHOOSE A SUBTLE STAINER

As you get older you lose the colour from your lips, so even if you prefer to wear nothing more than lip gloss or balm you should prime lips with a subtle stain first to enhance your natural colour.

LONG-LASTING LIPS

Long-lasting lipsticks that really stain lips are best avoided. They are hard to apply perfectly, will emphasize the shape and size of your lips and show every lip line that has formed around the mouth. Best to stick to neutral gloss and nude tints which will make the most of what you have.

SHEER LIGHTNESS

If you have a small mouth and thin lips, steer clear of dark, matt colours which will make your mouth look meaner, and visually accentuate the flesh-coloured wrinkles that form around the lips. Instead go for sheer, light colours of a similar shade to your natural lip colour.

MAKE TEETH WHITER

Choose your lipstick colour carefully; shades of purple or blue-based pinks can make teeth look whiter, while orangey browns will make them look yellowish.

CHOOSING A LIPSTICK

Don't wear make-up when you go to choose a new lipstick because then you can look at the true colour of your skin and lips and find a colour that suits your unmade-up skin tones.

PERFECT PARTY LIPS

When you're at a party and don't have time to keep re-touching lipstick, find one that has a waxy base which will stay put all evening, and will not bleed into the fine lines around your mouth.

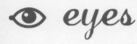

SWEEP IT UP

After you've applied foundation sweep a darker shade of bronzer or powder from the outside top edge of your eyebrow towards your hairline. This will give your eyes the illusion of being higher and wider.

NATURALLY SOFT AND SHEER

Soft, neutral shades will help to open up eyes, while dark moody ones can make them look smaller and deep set. Too much shimmer will settle into crease lines and reflect light, which will only draw attention to any crow's feet, so limit shimmer to the inner corner of the eyes.

SEMI-PERMANENT TIME SAVER

A non-surgical treatment, semi-permanent make-up is implanted into the skin using an infusion of organic or mineral pigments. Adding stronger definition to the eyelid can save time and give an "optical lift" to open up the eye. Consult a recommended professional.

LONG MAY IT LAST

If you want your eyeshadow to last all day, prime your eyelids with a thin layer of foundation before applying your eye colour. If you forgo shadow for a bare look, it will also help your eyelids blend in with the skin tone on the rest of your face, in which case using mascara will be necessary to give your eyes some definition.

HEAVY METAL MAGIC

To brighten dark eyes, dot a tiny smudge of silver metallic shadow on the inside corner of the eye, and it will give the effect of widening the eyes, and making them sparkle.

AFTERNOON CLEAN-UP

A cotton bud (swab) dipped in petroleum jelly or lip balm is a great way to clean up smudged eye make-up, thereby avoiding that bad mid-afternoon habit of washing everything off and reapplying – a sure-fire way to use up products twice as fast. Make sure you don't get any in your eyes!

TAPE FOR PERFECTION

Low-tack masking tape can safely create the perfect lines for precise liquid eyeliner. The trick is to cut a piece about 2.5 cm (1 in) long and peel it off the skin of your hand once or twice to lose a little of the stickiness. Then place at the desired angle on the corners of your eyes.

SHADOW FIXES

Keep your eyeliner in place, and reduce the need for constant reapplication, by patting dabs of black eyeshadow on top of it. This will stop your eyeliner smudging or bleeding and will keep your precious kohl stick lasting that bit longer.

REFRIGERATOR FRESH

Try keeping eye pencils, lipsticks and nail polishes in the refrigerator. This will stop them drying out and make them easier to apply. It should also prevent the tips of pencils and lipsticks from breaking off.

RETURN BAD ADVICE

If you buy a product on the advice of a counter assistant and then find it's not suitable or doesn't do what was promised, it's much easier to get a refund than buying "off the rack" in a pharmacy.

FINAL TOUCH

When you've finished making up your eyes, put a tiny spec of iridescent colourless shadow onto the centre of your eyelid near the lashes. This will pick up light and make eyes look wider and less hooded than they really are.

GO ALL THE WAY

Whether you choose to use a smudgy soft eyeliner pencil or a liquid liner, always draw across the whole length of the upper eye. Just covering half of the top lid will make your eyes look smaller and more close set.

 # mascara

CREATE A CURL

Eyelash curlers really do help to open up your eyes, which can become less accentuated with age, and there seems to be little difference between the cheapest and more expensive ones. Curl your eyelashes before you apply mascara as you are less likely to create clumps.

BROWN FOR BLONDES

If you are fair skinned and have natural or highlighted blonde hair, lay off the heavy black mascara, as it will look unnatural and harsh. Blondes should always choose dark brown mascara, which suits their colouring much better.

NO-MASCARA LASHES

If you always end up with mascara running down your face by the end of the evening, think about having your lashes tinted and permed. Dark, curly lashes without layers of cloggy mascara will draw attention to your eyes in the best possible way.

NO MORE CLOGGING

Sweep your mascara brush upwards in a generous curve to make lashes appear longer and thicker, but only brush the ends of the lashes and keep it away from the roots. Too much thick mascara around the base of the lashes will make eyes look small and narrow.

FLIRTY EYELASH EXTENSIONS

As hair starts to thin, some people notice their eyelashes fading, dropping out and almost disappearing. Some salons now offer a process that adds long, thick lashes to your own with a non-toxic bonding process. Synthetic lashes are individually attached to each natural eyelash to offer fantastic length and colour, and a fluttery, flirty effect. It is very important, however, to follow the strict care guidelines that go with them.

GO FOR LENGTH

If you tint your lashes to save time on making up with mascara, always use a clear gel mascara wand over the top. It contains tiny fibres that lengthen your lashes, and make them look longer than they really are.

GO WIDE

Concentrate mascara application on the outside of the eye – this will help to widen eyes and bring attention to the curved edges, making them appear more alluring.

KEEP IT UP TOP

Always use less mascara on your lower lashes; this will naturally "lift" your eyes. Too much on lower lashes can make eyes look droopy.

ONE COAT AT A TIME

Apply one coat of mascara carefully and wait for it to dry before considering a second one – you may only need one application. This way, you'll avoid clogging.

DOUBLE-UP MASCARA AS LINER

For a quick but glamorous look when you only have a limited bag
of make-up, use a loaded-up black mascara wand at the base of
the lower lashes to create a flattering line along the lower eye. This
quick trick will accentuate and open up the eye when you are caught
without your usual eye pencil.

LASH-EXTENSION MASCARA

Ageing can leave you with shorter and lighter-coloured lashes. Find a
mascara that has copper peptides listed in the ingredients; it is known
to enrich hair follicles and make lashes longer.

WEAR LIGHT LAYERS

Three or four coats of thinly applied mascara are more alluring and
natural-looking than one or two clumpy applications. When it comes
to eyelashes, the thinner the better!

LUBRICATE YOUR LASHES

Rub Vaseline, baby oil or eyelash conditioner into eyelashes overnight
(do this with your eyes closed). This will help keep your lashes
conditioned and prevent any breakage of the ends.

FAKE IT

You can enhance the length of your natural lashes without ending
up looking like a drag queen if you alternate the length of the fakes.
Apply short and medium-sized fake lashes side by side for a special
eye-opening party face.

CULL OLD MASCARA

If you've had your mascara for more than three or four months, it's
time to throw it out and get a new one. Over this time, the colour will
dry out and prevent you being able to put on smooth, even coats.

WARM UP MASCARA

If your mascara thickens when it reaches the end of the tube, place
the sealed tube in warm water for a few minutes to help make the
mascara thinner.

SPURN THE CHURN

Don't churn your mascara wand around in the mascara vial, it could introduce air and make it clog. A simple in-and-out movement will do, and keep the top on whenever it's not in use.

BE STILL

Don't be tempted to apply mascara or liner if you're on the move, in a car or on a train, however late you are. It's impossible to make an even job of it, however steady your hand.

TRIM YOUR FALSIES

Trim false eyelashes before you apply them to mimic the natural shape of your eyelashes and to define your eyes. Make the outer edges longer for eye-widening results.

BRUSH AWAY CLOGS

If you don't have a mascara comb to hand, get rid of nasty looking clogs by following your mascara application with a quick brush through with an old, washed-and-dried mascara wand.

DON'T ADD WATER

Never add water or other liquid to mascara to keep it from drying out, as this can cause the preservative to become diluted and therefore offer less protection against germs and bacteria.

PREVENT OVERLOAD

When you first buy mascara it's thinner and more liquid, which means it goes on heavier. To avoid over-doing it, and to ensure a lighter covering, allow the wand to dry for a few seconds in the air before you apply.

MONOGAMOUS MASCARA

Never share mascara – this is the most common way to pass on eye infections such as conjunctivitis. Also don't use the same mascara if you've just had an eye infection, which could re-introduce the infection or affect the other eye.

WASH BEFORE THE WAND

Always wash your hands before applying mascara to cut down the risk of passing on bacteria with your hands, especially if you're one of those people who uses their hands to touch their eye area while they apply.

GET THE WIGGLES

When applying mascara, wiggle your wand on the base of the lashes. It's the mascara near the roots – not the tips – that gives the illusion of length and thickness.

STROKE IT ON

For the smoothest results, stroke on colour in smooth strokes, from root to tip and in an upward motion. Avoid side-to-side movements, which can apply it too thickly.

PLUM IT UP

For a different look on dark lashes, go for a top coat of plum mascara to bring out the colour of dark hair and eyes. Applying it over black is an excellent evening option.

WORK THE WAND

First, apply mascara to the middle and inner lashes using upward strokes, then concentrate on the outer lashes, sweeping out at a 45-degree angle to enhance the outer edge of the eye.

GET RIDGES

Choosing a mascara applicator with ridges rather than bristles can help avoid clogs by ensuring an even coating. Mascara can get stuck in bristles, which are then passed on to your lashes.

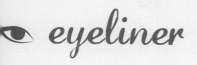 # eyeliner

KEEP SPARKLE SUBTLE

For subtle sparkle, choose an eyeliner with some added glitter that will give you a little bit of extra glamour. Don't be tempted to use other sparkly products on your eyes at the same time though.

FLATTEN OUT ROUND EYES

Make like a cat by flattening round eyes. Apply a liner only to the top lashes from the inner to the outer corners of the eye to give it a more elongated appearance.

DON'T BE BLUNT

Sharpen your eye pencil every time you use it. This prevents eye bacteria building up on the round, blunt end, which could spread to other parts of your eyes. It will also help you achieve high definition as blunt ends are much harder to control.

HOT SMOKE

Create a smoky evening look by running your eye pencil under hot water before you apply it for a deeper, smudgy look.

MODERNIZE YOUR EYES

Instead of using eyeliner for daily make-up, use powder eyeshadow applied with a very narrow brush to give a smoky, modern appearance to the edge of eyes. Smudge further if necessary with a larger brush. Alternatively, use the powder wet for a sharper line of colour.

SMOKE IT OUT

For a natural smoky look, whatever colour your eyeliner pencil is, smudge it in tiny circular motions that will provide you with a naturally blended line.

BE A KOHL KITTEN

Create that classic sex kitten effect on the eyes by lining the top and bottom lash lines to the outer corners in a classic black kohl pencil. Set this off with a few lashings of curl-enhancing mascara.

STAY OUTSIDE

Unless you're blessed with almond-shaped eyes, stick to using eyeliner on the outside rather than inside the lash line. Applying it inside will make your peepers seem smaller and dull their colour.

LINE UP THE BROWN

For paler skins, light browns and taupe eyeliners work best because they enhance the natural tones of the eye without overpowering the surrounding skin.

IT'S COOL TO BE SHARP

Eyeliners will sharpen better after a few hours in the fridge – the cold makes the ends firmer and less prone to stickiness. Let them warm up to room temperature before you use them or they'll be too hard.

KEEP LIQUID THIN

Liquid eyeliners are great for a defined evening look, but don't extend the line beyond the natural corner of the eye and keep it thin for the most glamorous look. If you have trouble keeping steady, try making three dashes – at the inner, middle and outer corners, then joining them up.

HIDE EYE CIRCLES

To draw attention away from under-eye bags or circles, avoid applying eyeliner or mascara to lower lashes, which could draw attention downward instead of up.

WIDEN WITH WHITE

To give your eyes the appearance of being wider set, line the inside of the bottom rim of your eyes with a soft white eyeliner pencil. This will also give you a fresher, younger look.

GO FOR THE TILT

To apply liner to your upper lash line, tip your head back and look down into a mirror. Rest a slightly blunted pencil tip on the lash line and push between your lashes, from inside to outside.

COOL FOR KOHL

Kohl pencils are ideal for summer days because they give a slightly waxy, soft look, which is simple and natural. For a clean look, use thin kohl pencils rather than crayons, which can be messier.

FEATHER IT WELL

Avoid sharp, hard lines around your eyes, which looks dated and obvious, by feathering eyeliner and blending it with a little powder for a smoky look.

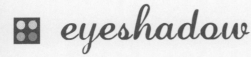 eyeshadow

KEEP IT ALL UP TOP
If you often find your eyes look puffy underneath, keep make-up focused on the top of the lid. Avoid under-eye mascara if you're puffy because it tends to smudge, and shade only the upper eyes to make them look more open.

LESS SHADOW, BETTER RESULTS
Use eyeshadows sparingly, as eyelids become wrinkled and hooded as we age, and a heavy-handed application of shadow will lie in creases along the wrinkles.

SHADOW IS SOFTER
A smudgy eyeshadow line can be more flattering than a hard sweep of eyeliner. Blend the outer edges to create a softer look, which doesn't draw so much attention to the fine lines and creases around the eyes. Use a shadow powder and eyeliner brush rather than a pencil to push the shadow into the lash line.

CREAM SHADOW NOT POWDER
Because the skin on our eyelids becomes dry and thin as we age, choose a cream eyeshadow in preference to a powder one, as it will last longer on the eyelid.

BE A ONE-TRICK WONDER
As a general rule, let your eyes or your lips do the talking – not both. This doesn't mean neglecting either area, just plump for a more natural look for one and use stronger make-up on the other. Usually you will want to concentrate on your best feature.

GLOW FOR GOLD
Give eyes a gorgeous glistening glow for summer by dusting a shimmer golden bronzer or loose gold dust over eyelids and cheekbones. To add intensity, highlight the outer corners of your eyes with a darker copper or brown eyeshadow.

COMPLEMENT, DON'T COLOUR

The purpose of eyeshadow is to shape and accentuate the eye, not
colour it. Even if you're going bright, choose tones that accentuate
your natural shades.

DAYLIGHT IS BRIGHT ENOUGH

Steer clear of bright eyeshadow or coloured mascara in the daytime
because harsh sunlight can make the colours appear even brighter,
washing out your face and eyes. Leave the bright colours for creating
dazzling looks in the evening.

GET BRAND SAVVY

If you're using two shades of powdered eyeshadow, use the same
brand, as they are more likely to be of the same formula, thus easier
to blend with each other.

SPARKLE IT UP WITH GOLD AND BRONZE

For evenings, there are several illuminating, loose and pressed
powders on the market, which add a bit of sparkle with both gold and
bronze flecked effects.

KEEP IT NEUTRAL

Do use flattering neutrals to contour and highlight your eyes for a
timeless daytime look that will last. For eyeliners, stick to classic
colours like black, navy or brown.

LIGHTEN YOUR INNER CORNERS

Often the inner corner of your eye, near the nose, is the darkest
part and can drag down your whole face. If you use a slightly lighter
shadow or eye pencil on this area, it will bring it out of the dark and
help your eyes look bigger, too.

LOOK LIVELY

For sparkling whites of eyes, go for cooler shades near the corner of
the eyes, where the colour is nearest the eyeball. Avoid yellows and
reds in this area, which can make your eyes look sickly.

GREEN UP THE BLUE

If you have blue eyes, enhance their natural colour with a subtle green eyeshadow rather than blue – it will bring out the blue eye colour without being overpowering.

TOUCH IT UP

If you're in a hurry, add extra touches of cream or gel-type eyeshadow with the tip of your middle finger. Just a dot of the product, applied lightly, should work just fine.

CREAMS INCREASE CREASES

Lightly powder lids before eyeshadow to keep them crease-proof longer. If you're prone to creasing, avoid cream colours in favour of silky powders.

SOFTEN UP FROGGY EYES

If you have large, prominent eyes, do not use loud or bright colours, which will over-emphasize their fullness. Go for soft shades and neutrals instead.

FOIL SPILLS

Apply a dusting of loose powder directly under-eye area before you apply your eyeshadow. Afterwards, whisk away the powder from under your eyes with a brush and it will take eyeshadow fallout with it.

DON'T OVERDO THE SHIMMER

Be careful with shimmery products, especially on your eyelids, as they tend to collect in the creases. They are best left for evening, where they won't have to hold the look for as long.

BRING EYES OUT WITH LIGHT

On deep-set eyes, choose shadow colours that are on the light side of the colour spectrum, particularly on the bit of lid directly above the eye, which will make them appear more prominent.

highlighters

DON'T SWEAT IT

Illuminators and highlighters are great for picking out areas you want
to highlight, but take care when applying them as a skin base or you
could end up looking as if you have a sweaty face. Mix a tiny amount
with your usual foundation for best results.

DOTS OF LIGHT

Dots of highlighter have a powerful illuminating effect. Apply a dot of
highlighter in the inner corners of the eyes, on the lips or on the tip of
the nose to add shine and definition to your face.

BE A RADIANT WOMAN

A perfect remedy for hungover skin, radiance boosters are applied
after moisturizer and before foundation, but they also work well when
patted over make-up for a quick, midday perk-up. They add instant
glow, making you appear more wide-awake and fresher.

BOOST WITH A SPRITZ

Spritzing rosewater or a water spray over make-up is an instant
reviver. It rehydrates skin and adds a natural glow, helping to get that
natural dewy look without adding any extra product.

GOLDEN GIRLS

Gold-based highlighters are great in the summer when applied on
top of bare skin or for darker complexions. In the cooler winter light,
however, choose the pink versions to give the same effect.

SHIMMER IT UP

Mixing a few drops of highlighter or shimmer lotion into liquid
foundation gives a subtle gleam, which you can use to highlight
areas such as cheekbones, eyebrows and the upper lip.

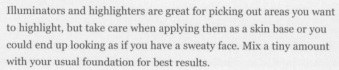

CHOOSE YOUR PRODUCT

Many highlighters and illuminators come as creams, balms,
multipurpose sticks and tubes for applying in specific areas or
blending in all over the face.

DON'T SHIMMER WITH DISCO GLITTER

For a versatile choice, choose a fine, loose powder shimmer that you
can apply with a blusher brush, not only on the face but also on the
shoulders, décolletage and legs.

LOOK WHERE THE LIGHT HITS

Apply highlighter on those areas that are directly hit by daylight, such
as the tops of the cheekbones and the temples. Stand in front of a
mirror in a bright light to test the best areas.

perfect smile

CONTRAST CONTROL

You can make your teeth look instantly brighter without expensive
whitening treatments by applying fake tan or bronzer to your face!

A ROOT SOLUTION

Radishes contain fluorine – a trace element that strengthens tooth
enamel. Try them sliced in salads and stir-fries.

LIP SERVICE

For a quick whitening boost use a blue-toned, glossy red lipstick. Avoid
orange and yellow tones as they can make teeth look yellow. Pale,
frosted shades tend to make your teeth look dull as do matte finishes.

MINTY FRESH

Why pay for a breath freshener that will give you minty breath when
fresh mint is easy to grow yourself? Make your own mouth spray by
pouring boiling water over fresh mint leaves and leaving overnight.
Decant into a sterilized spray bottle and add a tablespoon of vodka to
preserve. Store in the refrigerator.

UNPAID PROTECTION

If you're going to be drinking red wine or coffee, protect your teeth by coating them with a thin layer of petroleum jelly. The coating acts as a cheap but clever barrier to prevent staining.

AVOCADO BREATH

If the root of your bad breath is acid indigestion, a cheap and easy solution is to eat some avocado. This healthy fruit effectively boosts digestion, preventing food from sitting in your stomach for too long.

PEARLY APPEAL

Apples contain pectin, which can help to neutralize food odours. So the next time you have a spicy curry or garlicky dinner, have an apple for dessert.

BREATH OF SUNSHINE

Eat a handful of sunflower seeds and drink a glass of water to treat bad breath. This low-calorie snack doesn't contain sugar or foul-tasting sweetener unlike many store-bought breath-freshener mints.

ALL CREDIT TO THE CRUNCH

The credit crunch might be causing you headaches but crunchy foods such as fresh apples and celery naturally remove red wine, tea or coffee stains from the enamel of your teeth – at a fraction of the price of expensive stain-removing toothpastes.

BE FUSSY ABOUT FLUORIDE

Toothpaste containing fluoride is a wise investment. Fluoride kills bacteria and is also assimilated into the teeth, strengthening them and making them more resistant to decay.

AN APPLE A DAY KEEPS...

This inexpensive snack increases saliva secretion, which protects your teeth against cavities and decay. A post-dinner apple makes for an instant "brush", but never actually brush your teeth straight after eating fruit as the combination of scrubbing and fruit acid can wear away tooth enamel.

MILKY GOODNESS

To protect your teeth from decay eat plenty of low-fat live yogurt.
This budget snack is high in calcium, which helps to keep your teeth
cavity-free and is a natural bacteria fighter. Research also shows that
people who get enough calcium in their diet are less likely to develop
severe gum disease.

A CHEESY GRIN

Make a small slice of hard cheese part of your diet every other day.
Cheese helps to stop bacteria from growing in the mouth and prevents
cavities. Be careful not to overdo the amount as cheese is high in
unhealthy saturated fats!

STAIN-REMOVING STRAWBERRY

These clever berries have a natural bleaching effect on your teeth.
Simply wipe over teeth for a sparkling smile.

GET INTERDENTAL

If you have gappy teeth, bridges or implants, an interdental brush
is often better than floss for cleaning between the teeth and keeping
gums in the pink.

GET COLOUR CLEVER

To make teeth appear whiter, wear lipsticks in cool, bright hues (pink,
raspberry, plum) with a glossy finish.

CHOOSE CHLORHEXIDINE

Chlorhexidine is the best ingredient to beat inflamed gums or gum
disease. It is designed for short-term use and is available in special
mouthwashes.

DO LOVE YOUR TEETH

A great set of teeth will always make you look like a million dollars.
And remember, prevention is always cheaper – so instead of spending
money on whitening treatments, take good care of your teeth with
thorough brushing and daily flossing.

GINGER AWAY FUR

If you have a furry tongue, drink more water as dehydration is a major cause of this. If this doesn't work, try sucking on a piece of fresh ginger, which can help reduce bacteria in the mouth naturally.

BE NATURAL WITH SEAWEED

Seaweed as a food supplement is thought to keep teeth and gums healthy by getting rid of excess plaque, but don't stop brushing and flossing as well.

TEETH LOVE TEA

Tea contains polyphenols, which fight plaque-causing dental bacteria and ward off cavities, and makes it harder for bacteria to cling to your teeth. Green tea contains the highest amounts, but you'll still get plenty from a cheap cup of standard tea.

KISS AWAY YOUR DOUBLE CHIN

It takes 34 individual muscles to pucker up for a goodnight kiss, and the longer it goes on, the better the workout they'll get. Keep cheeks firm with regular kissing, and your partner will thank you, too!

DISCLOSE YOUR WEAKNESS

Two-thirds of people who brush their teeth twice a day leave plaque deposits behind. Chew a disclosing tablet after brushing and any remaining plaque will turn red, enabling you to spot and target your trouble spots.

SCRAPE YOUR TONGUE

Tongue scraping is a very important part of oral hygiene as it rids the mouth of bacteria that can lead to bad breath and plaque build-up that can also stain the teeth.

JOIN THE JET-SET

Dental water jets are designed to be used after flossing for additional cleaning and polishing. They can be useful for people with bridges, implants or gum disease.

GUM MASSAGE

Dentists recommend gentle gum massage to strengthen and firm gums, enhance blood flow to the area, fight gingivitis and prevent disease. You can use special gum brushes for this purpose, or massage the gums daily with your index finger – combine with a herbal gum wash or oil for added benefit.

INVEST IN LEMON ZEST

Whiten teeth naturally by brushing with grated lemon zest, a natural bleaching agent that will whiten teeth without damaging your gums.

KEEP GUMS IN THE PINK

Younger gums sit tight on teeth without gaps. To keep gums looking young and healthy avoid over-brushing or brushing too hard, which can contribute to gum recession, making you look older than your years.

ENLIST YOUR DENTIST

Use a whitening toothpaste once a week and, more importantly, visit your dentist every six months to have teeth cleaned, especially the gaps between them – it's a sure-fire way of looking more beautiful.

INSIDE-OUT BRIGHT

Internal bleaching places the bleaching product inside the tooth. The dentist will drill a hole in the tooth and put the product inside, sealing the hole with a temporary filling, and leaving the bleach inside the tooth. About a week later, the bleach is taken out, and the small hole filled.

KEEP SMILING

Nothing is more attractive than a woman with a happy smile. It makes you look young, fun and carefree, so don't save your smile for special occasions – do it every day.

VENEER IT WISELY

Veneers, with or without dental re-shaping, can bring uniformity to your smile. Thin porcelain veneers are bonded to your teeth, helping to disguise teeth that are misaligned, worn, chipped or discoloured. They are translucent, which makes them appear natural.

HOME TEETH WHITENING

Whiten your teeth at home with an over-the-counter gel and tooth tray. You will need to use this for several hours in the day or overnight and should see the maximum results in two or three weeks.

LASER AWAY STAINS

A bleaching system that uses a laser and a whitening gel, is a one-off treatment that gets immediate results. A laser light activates the gel and penetrates the enamel.

BRIGHTEN YOUR SMILE

Teeth-whitening procedures remove discolouration and staining, up to four shades lighter. Among the various techniques are chemical whitening, mild acid, abrasive, and laser whitening. A clinic procedure is followed by an at-home follow-up treatment. Not suitable for those with sensitive teeth and gums.

QUICK-TIME ORTHODONTICS

Straight, even teeth can make a huge difference to your appearance. Accelerated orthodontics can achieve straightening and overbite or underbite correction in three to eight months, rather than the traditional two or three years.

SCULPT UNSHAPELY TEETH

There are a variety of options for correcting misshapen teeth, available from dental aesthetics' clinics. Re-sculpting uses gentle abrasion to reshape individual teeth; veneers or laminates are thin porcelain shapes bonded to the teeth.

PROFIT AND FLOSS

Flossing is one of the most important parts of an oral hygiene routine – use dental floss, tape or wired flossers that can help get to those hard-to-reach areas.

HEALTHY GUMS

Poor oral hygiene will lead to gingivitis and eventually to teeth becoming loose and starting to separate. Daily plaque removal and thorough brushing with a fluoride toothpaste will help to maintain healthy teeth and gums.

GET A LIFT

Oralift is a new anti-ageing dental brace that works by slightly widening the gap between the teeth which forces the muscles in your face to change shape slightly, boosting blood flow and rejuvenating its appearance by reducing wrinkles.

facial exercise & massage

WOBBLY CHIN BE GONE

A quick-fix facial toner that can be repeated 20 times a day wherever you are is to push your lips tight together and make a wide grimace. Hold for 3 seconds and repeat, to contract lower facial muscles and tighten a wobbly chin.

PLUMP YOUR MOUTH WITH A BAND

Try a facial flex fitness device specifically for facial muscles. Just two minutes a day with a resistance band should improve circulation and skin firmness, and help to reduce double chins and a wrinkly jaw.

TIGHTEN UP FACIAL MUSCLES

Like a wobbly tummy, facial muscles need to be exercised on a regular basis to stop them becoming loose and flabby. A routine that takes just 10 minutes a day, and which can be done anywhere – on the bus, in the car or watching TV – will tighten up lazy skin.

PINCH TO RELIEVE STRESS

Many people hold stress in the area between the brows and in time vertical stress lines will develop here. When you feel your brow knit together with concentration or stress, take a moment to pinch the muscle here, working from the centre of the brow along the browline in each direction with a thumb and bent forefinger.

MASSAGE WITH A FRIEND

Regular facial massages don't have to mean an expensive trip to the salon – it is the action of gentle massage on the face that relaxes the muscles, stimulates the blood vessels under the skin and helps keep fine lines at bay.

GET YOUR FINGERS WORKING

Just a few minutes a day of fingertip massage can increase circulation in the face leaving your complexion revitalized and rigid frown lines less set. Age causes the connective tissue to become less supple, so massage must be delicate and fingers not probe too deeply. Try simply tapping two fingers from beside the mouth to along the jawline to stimulate circulation and promote glow.

WAKE UP YOUR FACE

In the morning the face can look pale and puffy because of the natural nocturnal slow-down in the body. When putting on your moisturizer, take the opportunity to gently massage all the muscles in the face to waken up the lymphatic system and jumpstart the circulation.

tools of the trade

LIGHT IT UP

If you have a habit of overdoing your make-up, make sure you're using a mirror with a powerful enough light. Overdone cheeks or foundation "tide marks" are common mistakes for people who lack voltage.

NO-NO TO NYLON

In most cases use natural bristles rather than nylon or other synthetics, which are stiff and can scratch the face. Most make-up artists prefer natural hair as it blends softly and smoothly.

SIZE IT UP

For the most effective application, choose make-up brushes that match the size of the area they are to be used on. Brushes for eyelids will be smaller than cheek brushes.

CULL YOUR MAKE-UP BAG

Make-up might rarely come with use-by dates, but often it's just like food – leave it too long and it will go off. Don't keep lipsticks for more than two years, foundation for more than a year or sunscreen for more than six months to be super-safe.

LOOK WHERE YOU'RE GOING

Low-level-lighting can completely alter a look. Whatever light you're going to be seen in, try to make-up in a similar light or at least take the time to check how your make-up looks in similar conditions. To avoid mistakes use a make-up mirror that has several light options for day and night, and cool and warm lighting.

FLUFF YOUR LINES

Invest in a large, fluffy brush for applying cheek colour – this will ensure soft, natural-looking lines when you apply it.

KEEP IT DARK AND COOL

Because of the preservatives and active ingredients they contain, all make-up products will last longer and stay more effective if they are kept away from heat sources and direct sunlight. The best place to keep them is in a drawer, fridge or cupboard away from the light.

BRUSH UP YOUR EYES

Don't be tempted to use fingers to apply eyeshadow – a natural-fibre brush is essential for accurate blending and a professional, well-applied look. Avoid nylon brushes, which will only spread colour around rather than shade the eye.

GET SHORTY

Most make-up brushes are too long to fit into a small make-up bag. Try getting travel size versions or brushes that twist up from the base.

BLEND IT WELL

Everyone needs a blending brush – this should be different from the one you use to apply your eyeshadow, which gets covered in the product. Blending brushes should be soft and clean, and used to give make-up a more natural look.

WALKING THE THIN LINE

Invest in a thin, flat brush that can be used to apply shaped lines and contours to eyeshadow and highlighter. Use the brush to apply the right amount, then blend with a clean brush to create a professional look.

WASH THOROUGHLY

Wash your make-up brushes in soapy water at least every three months to keep them clean and clog-free. If someone else uses your brushes, wash them thoroughly before you use them again or you risk introducing bacteria into your make-up. Cosmetic sponges and applicators should be washed once a week. Rinse them well and dry flat.

DON'T GET STUCK IN

Try not to stick your fingers in the pot if you can help it, as this increases the chances of introducing unwanted bacteria into the product. Use a clean plastic spatula or a spoon instead.

COLLECT LIKE A PRO

One of the things that sets make-up artists apart is their collection of brushes. Book a make-up lesson and see which brushes they use to do your make-up, then ask them to suggestion an essential at-home kit.

VIVE LA DIFFERENCE

There is nothing more frustrating than trying to apply a light shade and getting a darker smudge as a result of the last colour you used with the same brush. Keep brushes for dark and light shades separate.

MILD BENEFIT

To avoid irritation, use a daily cleanser or a mild washing-up liquid to wash your brushes. These are more gentle alternatives to the specially formulated brush cleaners that can be harsh and cause skin reactions.

GET BACK IN SHAPE

Reshape your brushes after washing, laying them out flat and letting them dry naturally before reusing them. If the bristles frizz and shed, it's time to buy new ones as there's no way to recondition the brushes once they are worn out. Keep an eye on the shape, too – each brush has a specific shape for an application purpose and once this deteriorates you will not get good results.

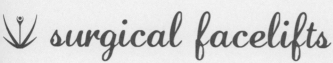 # surgical facelifts

BETTER BROW LIFTS

Keyhole surgery is on the increase to rejuvenate the forehead and lift the eyebrows. Ageing causes the brows to droop and look tired, which causes horizontal creases in the forehead. These days brow lifts involve short incisions, 1cm (½ inch) long, that are hidden within the scalp, resulting in a fresher, more open appearance in the upper third of the face.

EARLY 40S FACELIFT

The most common procedures for people in this age group who want tightening in the face are performed with a shorter scar. The scar in front of the ear is a normal procedure, but behind the ear the scar is small and does not extend up into the scalp.

FACE UP TO A FACELIFT

There are several types that can be done to rejuvenate an ageing face, and the scars are designed to be well hidden. Skin at the temples, cheeks, and neck is tightened upwards and backwards, and the layer of muscle tissue which lies underneath the skin (SMAS layer) is also treated in a similar way.

KNOW YOUR ZONES

In plastic surgery, the face is divided into three important horizontal zones, each one considered differently. The first is from the brows to the hairline where deep forehead furrows and brow lifts are done; the second is the eyelid to cheek area where crow's feet, hooded lids and under-eye bags manifest; and the third is the lower face and neck area. Most facelifts target zones 1 and 2, as only subtle differences can be made to zone 3.

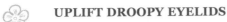

UPLIFT DROOPY EYELIDS

Puffy, tired-looking eyes are usually caused by a combination of loose skin and excess fat. Common problems of hooded eyes and bags can all be solved with eyelid surgery (blepharoplasty), which involves operating on the eyelid itself or removing and adjusting excess skin and fat.

A BRAND NEW NECKLINE

Most neck lifts are performed simultaneously to a deep plane facelift, the aim being to eliminate vertical folds in the neck, to tighten the skin, and to reduce excess fat. The incisions are usually the same as for a facelift although a small cut under the chin, known as a platysmaplasty, may be required.

A LONGER-LASTING LIFT

Surgeons need to lift a deeper layer of skin to provide a longer-lasting result. By removing the soft tissues to which the muscles are attached (SMAS) and tightening them, or by lifting up a portion of the SMAS itself, it is possible to treat saggy jowls and redefine the neck.

A QUICK LIFT

The MACS lift (minimal access cranial suspension) is good for patients with mild skin sagging, but no heavy folds around the neck. Permanent sutures are used to lift the soft facial tissue and suspend them in a more youthful position. There is a relatively quick recovery time, and a short scar behind the ears.

THE FAT-INJECTION FACELIFT

Known as the Volumetric facelift, volume can be added to restore a youthful appearance. Fat from your own body can be injected into the face to plump up gauntness, and cheek tissue can be repositioned to the site it occupied before gravity produced its downward drift.

THE CUTANEOUS CUT

One of the first types of facelift that has been performed for many years, this relies on lifting the upper layer of skin only. Facial improvement occurs by lifting skin backwards and upwards, but there is no improvement to deeper facial muscles.

 facial peels

PHENOL PEEL DOWNTIME

A full-face deep facial peel can take a couple of hours to perform and should always be done by a qualified dermatologist. The treatment can leave you in bandages for several days and looking red and sore for weeks, but severe wrinkling around the mouth and eyes will be dramatically improved and the benefits of the fresh new skin that emerges are long lasting.

SKIN RESURFACING

Effective techniques in skin resurfacing, designed to even out the surface and reduce pigmentation, can now be performed in your lunch hour at the beauty salon. The improvements can seem miraculous, but the treatments can be invasive and are not without risk, so you should not undergo any cosmetic procedure without good research.

OPERATION CROW'S FEET

A medium peel using trichloroacetic acid (TCA) removes the epidermis and the upper layers of the dermis, penetrates more deeply than AHAs, and requires a recovery time of about a week. Surface wrinkles, crow's feet, minor scarring and small pre-cancerous moles are all suitable for this treatment.

A SUPERFICIAL LIGHT PEEL

Treatments that use alphahydroxy acids (AHAs) are light, and will only remove the upper layer of skin. A series of peels is usually recommended, which will result in softer skin and the stimulation of cell and collagen production.

PEEL AWAY OLD SKIN

A chemical peel is simply an aggressive form of exfoliation that removes the top layer of the epidermis and all the flaws with it. The type of solution applied to the face, and the amount of time it stays on for, all determine how deep the peel is and how good the results are.

DRYING-OUT SPOTS

A light glycolic acid peel will help to dry out patches of adult acne, dislodge blackheads and reduce shallow scarring, leaving your complexion brighter and softer. It makes skin more sensitive to UV radiation, so you will always need to use a non-irritating sun block.

TARGET SPECIFIC PROBLEMS

A full facial dermabrasion treatment will incur a lot of swelling and skin can look sore for up to 12 weeks, but the treatment is very useful for targeting trouble spots like specific scars or deep-set lines around the mouth.

RESURFACE THE EXTREMITIES

Light and medium peels can also be performed on the hands and the neck area to reduce visible scars and wrinkles, and help stimulate the production of new skin cells.

NON-CHEMICAL PEELS

Microdermabrasion uses a high-powered combination of force plus suction to remove a very thin layer of skin, and leaves only the most superficial wounds. Finely ground aluminium oxide or sodium crystals are blasted onto the skin, sloughing off the top layer and leaving a fresh new layer underneath.

SAND BLASTING

More aggressive than microdermabrasion or chemical peels, this procedure requires a specialist to "sand" off the top layer of skin using a hand-held electrical device. When the new skin grows back it will be smoother, less wrinkled, and with all signs of age spots or scarring reduced.

DEEPER EXFOLIATION NEEDS A HIGH DOSE

Phenol peels are peels with high concentrated solutions of acid, which are used to remove the epidermis and a large part of the dermis. As a treatment for deep facial wrinkles, areas of blotchy or sun-damaged skin and cancerous growths, phenol peels have proved to be very successful.

BETAHYDROXY ACID PEELS

A good alternative to an AHA peel, the betahydroxy peel has been found to be less irritating to the skin. As the salicylic acid it involves is fat-soluble, the peel can penetrate oil-plugged pores and so is good for people with active acne. Treatment may leave you with peeling skin for a few days, but it will remove blemishes and improve pigmentation.

cosmetic fillers & relaxers

PLUMP WITH COLLAGEN
Derived from bovine collagen (from cattle specifically reared for the purpose) this is one of the most commonly used fillers made to plump out laughter lines around the eyes and turn thin lips into voluptuous ones.

SALINE KISSES
Saline lip implants are inserted through tiny incisions along lip borders and then inflated with salt water, resulting in smooth and also bigger lips.

LIP PLUMP
For a temporary lip implant and for people who cannot tolerate collagen, these hyaluronic acid gels are used with great success because they have the same chemical and molecular structure as an enzyme present in humans that helps keep skin moist and elastic.

FILL OUT WITH FAT TRANSFERS
Autolgous fat transplantation plumps up skin using your own fat that has been liposuctioned from your thighs or abdomen. This can be used for deep lines, lip augmentation and acne scars.

NATURAL ALTERNATIVES FOR LAUGHTER LINES
Isologen and Autologen are two natural fillers made from your own skin cells that have been previously removed and allowed to incubate in test tubes until they produce collagen. There is no chance of an allergic reaction and the injected treatment should last up to two years.

REMODEL WITH RADIO FREQUENCY

Skin tightening the jowly bits of the cheek that hang down below the jawline in ugly little bulges is now possible with a non-surgical procedure that involves radiofrequency remodeling. It contracts the skin that has stretched, giving it a lift and reducing the size of the jowls.

FILL THOSE WRINKLES

The technology to fill and reduce wrinkles is moving so quickly there are now many different types of filler available. Synthetic and natural, injectable and non-injectable, permanent and temporary, all basically perform the same function, which is to plump up the skin and create a more youthful appearance.

SOFTFORM IMPLANTS

This synthetic hollow tube implant is used for smile lines around the mouth and frown lines, as well as to boost ageing lips. It is implanted beneath the skin and your own body's fibrous tissue grows through it, helping to keep the implant in place.

SUPER GEL FILLS FACIAL LINES

A manmade filler called Outline is being used to plump out the lines that form from nose to mouth. Made from tiny positively charged spheres, it attracts negatively charged molecules like a magnet, and instantly becomes part of your skin tissue. Results are instantaneous and it can last for five years.

THE FACIAL FILLER DERMOLOGEN

Made from donor human cadaver skin, this treatment does not usually cause an allergic reaction, and is just injected into the area being treated, usually for lip augmentation and to plump out laughter lines. It lasts longer than collagen, probably about six months, before the implant is absorbed into the body.

BANISH LINES WITH BOTOX

Botox injections containing the botulinum toxin have revolutionized the anti-ageing program for the face. A tiny amount of the poison is injected into the skin and temporarily paralyzes the muscles, which can no longer make the same expression so lines are gradually smoothed and softened from lack of use. The areas it treats best are lines on the forehead and between the brows and crow's feet.

COMPUTERIZED FACELIFT

The science of Super TNS (Trophic Neuromuscular Stimulation) is designed to stimulate the foundation muscles of the face and body. The procedure will make skin look younger because of increased blood circulation, as well as enhancing tissue elasticity and lessening laughter and frown lines.

RESULTS WITH ARTECOLL

This filler combines bovine collagen with inert microscopic plastic "beads" (less than the diameter of human hair), which become encapsulated by the body's own collagen, and therefore stay in place. It is used for lip enhancement, deeper wrinkles and soft facial scars.

A SAFETOX ALTERNATIVE

Safetox is an adhesive patch fixed to the forehead and worn with a plastic headband that releases electronic impulses onto the frown lines on your face. Safetox inhibits the muscles that create wrinkles; it activates and relaxes them, creating the appearance of a youthful and radiant face.

TYPE A TOXIN

The most potent and commonly used type of botulinum toxin is type A. Because the toxin attaches itself to the muscle where it was injected, it cannot travel around the body and so cannot cause permanent damage. The effects should last for 3–6 months, by which time the body will naturally have destroyed the toxin.

BLOCK LINES WITH MYOBLOC

If your body has natural resistance to the botulinum toxin or you find it not strong enough to do the job, there is a larger dose called Myobloc which is a botulinum toxin type B. The effects are a little more immediate and results may last a little longer.

BOYS MAKE COSMODERM

Scientists have been able to isolate and then replicate the collagen-producing cells found in newborn infant boys after circumcision. These can be injected into the skin to treat fine lines and wrinkles.

BETTER THAN BOTOX

A toxin called Xeomin, which works in the same way as Botox, is thought to have less chances of an allergic reaction because it doesn't contain the lab-produced foreign protein cells that are used as a carrier – so look out for this alternative wrinkle-relaxer.

NEW GENERATION RADIANCE

Radiance (also known as Radiesse), a next-generation cosmetic filler, is an injectable paste made from a substance found in human bones and teeth. It can be used to fill laughter lines and folds, as well as being injected into lips to give a fuller pout.

FILLERS TO LOOK FOR

Argiform, Dermalive and polyactic acid are all synthetic fillers that have been developed to inject safely into the face where wrinkles, folds and depression lines have formed over the years due to natural loss of moisture. They restore volume and leave the face looking smoother.

RESTYLE WITH RESTYLANE

This dermal filler is made from hyaluronic acid that is derived from skin tissue and has been used in more than 3 million treatments. It restores volume to the skin, giving a smoother, more youthful appearance.

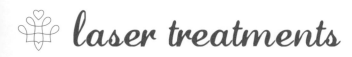

laser treatments

WHICH AREA TO TREAT?

For smoothing away wrinkles and resurfacing rough skin, lasers are best suited for three target areas of the face – the forehead and between the brows; the under-eye area extending to the crow's feet; and around the mouth.

ZAP THOSE SPIDER VEINS

Treat tiny spider veins on your face with Intense Pulsed Light laser. This pain-free and non-invasive treatment sends light pulses into the cells causing the vein to collapse and then dissolve.

LUNCHTIME TREATMENTS

A 15-minute treatment using the N-Lite laser, which uses a specific yellow laser light to reduce wrinkles around the eyes and stimulate the growth of collagen, will leave your skin tingling, but you can put on make-up and go back to work straight away.

LASER LIGHT TO NEW SKIN

Fractional lasers such as Fraxel can resurface the skin in a non-aggressive way, making it softer, smoother and tighter. Using light sources that can stimulate collagen production and improve the appearance of fine lines, wrinkles, acne scars and age spots, there is no pain and the redness only lasts for 2–3 days.

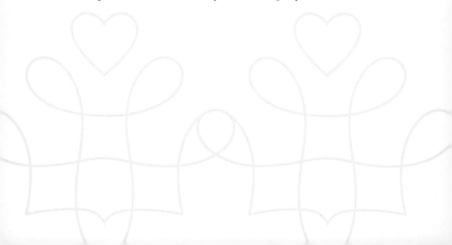

ABLATIVE LASER TREATMENT

There are 3 types of ablative lasers used for resurfacing the skin:
carbon dioxide (CO_2), erbium (Er: YAG); and the long-pulsed erbium
(YAG). A qualified dermatologist will select the most appropriate
treatment for you, but all focus laser energy on damaged surface
layers and vaporize them, allowing collagen regeneration and new
fresh smooth skin to grow.

MAGICAL LIGHT BEAMS

Laser treatments do not destroy outer tissue as they penetrate
through to the layers beneath the epidermis to boost collagen
production and improve skin texture giving it a tighter and plumper
appearance. The process is gradual and you will need multiple
sessions to see results.

NON-ABLATIVE LASER TREATMENT

Less intense than ablative treatments, they work by stimulating new
collagen production in the dermis, and cause skin contraction and
tightening. The treatment essentially works by treating wrinkles from
the inside out, rather than removing them from the outside.

REJUVENATE WITH LASER

Thought to be one of the safest forms of cosmetic surgery, laser
peeling offers more control in the depth of penetration and degree of
precision for resurfacing problem areas of wrinkles around lips and
eyes and specific scarring.

Haircare & Styling

DISCOVER THE PERFECT HAIRCARE routine, how to enhance the beauty of your hair, the cuts that suit your face shape and the colours that work for your skin tone. In these pages you will also find just-left-the-salon styling techniques, how to get the best blow-dry, and the products and tools to use for a fantastic finish. There are also solutions for troublesome problems such as thinning, grey, greasy, polluted or frizzy hair.

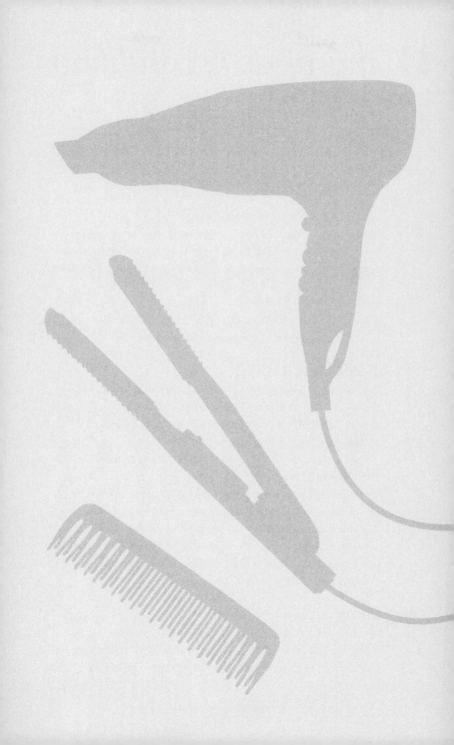

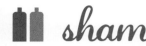 shampoo & condition

WASH THE ROOTS, NOT THE ENDS

When shampooing, concentrate on the roots, not the ends, of the hair – this will clean the greasiest sebum-producing area without stripping the drier parts. Don't worry about hair not being clean – the shampoo will cleanse the length of the hair as it rinses out.

GET HANDY WITH SHAMPOO

Instead of squeezing shampoo directly onto the top of the head, ensure even coverage by spreading it over your palms first, working it into a light lather and using your fingers to massage it evenly over the scalp.

WORK OUT KNOTS

Thoroughly brush your hair before you wash it – wet hair is much more fragile, so brushing it can cause splits and tears.

WASH YOUR HAIR

The best way to wash hair extensions is to soak them in cold water to which a capful of very mild shampoo has been added. Swish them around and then rinse in cool water. Let your extensions air-dry naturally and avoid heat products.

BUY THE BEST

Cheap shampoos are harsh detergents that are not formulated for the specific needs of your hair. They may contain drying alcohols or resins. Choose the best brand you can afford and buy for your needs – coloured, dry, fine, strengthening, and so on. These have ingredients such as antioxidants, vitamins, sun filters and penetrating strengtheners and moisturizers.

CONDITIONER FOR ALL

All hair needs a conditioner every time you shampoo. For very fine hair, use a light oil-free variety on the ends of the hair only. Stronger hair may need a leave-in conditioner as well as a rinse-out one.

SAVE YOUR TIME

All standard conditioners stop working after 30 minutes, so do not leave it on for longer in the belief that you will get greater benefits. For a deep condition, buy a separate conditioner or mask for the purpose – these contain moisturizers and vegetable proteins designed to penetrate into the hair shaft.

PILE ON THE MAYO

Many commercially bought cholesterol hair conditioners contain alcohol, the very thing that dries out hair. Instead of using one of these, massage a handful of mayonnaise into dry hair and wrap in plastic food wrap for ten minutes to boost moisture.

BANISH BUILD-UP

One of the major causes of problem hair is product build-up, which can be caused by using too much mousse, gel or spray, and not rinsing thoroughly enough. If necessary, shampoo twice to get really clean and always rinse more than you think you need it.

GET YOUR PRODUCTS RIGHT

Experiment with shampoos and conditioners until you find one that suits your hair and alternate them with another variety every few months to ensure the ingredients are working to their best ability and your hair's not "getting used" to them.

BE PREPARED

If you have a big event to prepare for and you're going to be short of time, or your hair will require styling, wash it the night before and it will be more manageable when you come to style it the next day.

BEAUTY AND THE BEAST

Bull's semen is the latest haircare treatment used to provide pure protein for dry, coarse hair. The intense conditioner, which also contains the root of the protein-rich plant katera, is massaged into the hair which is then treated with a steamer. This allows the product to penetrate deep into the hair before it is washed off, leaving soft and shiny locks.

WET IT DOWN

Make sure your hair is completely soaking wet before shampooing. Leave it under the shower for at least a full minute. You will need less shampoo and washing will be much easier.

CUT DOWN ON SHAMPOO

For the shiniest hair you've ever had, halve the amount of shampoo you use (a dessertspoon full should be enough for all but the longest hair) and double the amount of time you spend rinsing.

DEEP CONDITION

If your hair is bleached, give yourself a deep-conditioning treatment once a week to preserve as much moisture as possible in the dehydrated hair shaft and prevent bleach damage spreading through the hair.

SHINE UP WITH BEER

To give hair a really shiny finish and greater manageability, hairdressers recommend rinsing it in beer, which imparts a luscious, rich shine to the hair follicle. Rinse through with water afterwards to avoid smelling like a brewery!

CARROT-TOP CONDITIONER

Instead of buying a conditioner formulated for oily hair, simply massage finely grated carrots into your wet hair for 15 minutes before rinsing.

GET IN A LATHER

Don't worry about overwashing your hair if you do it every day or every other day. According to the experts, the more hair is shampooed, the better it responds to treatments. It is exposed to the same environment as the rest of your body, so needs to be cleaned just as much as your skin.

HEALTH CHECK

Our skin and hair both reflect the overall state of our health, so if your hair looks dull and unhealthy you need to check your nutritional intake. EFAs (essential fatty acids) are essential for glossy, vibrant hair, while zinc will help promote regrowth.

THE RIGHT SHAMPOO

If your hair has started to look dull, check the pH balance of your shampoo. The scalp's natural pH is between 4 and 6, but many shampoos are alkaline which can make hair dull and unhealthy-looking.

KEEP REGULAR APPOINTMENTS

Find a stylist you like and can trust to talk things through, and discuss what is possible with your hair type and texture. Make regular appointments every 6–8 weeks for a trim and to keep your colour touched up and get an intensive conditioning treatment.

CONDITION WITH CARE

Some leave-in conditioners are unsuitable for fine hair. They coat the hair to protect it, but they can weigh it down and make it dull and greasy and very difficult to style. Wash-out conditioners generally suit all hair types better.

SUPER SHINE

For extra shiny hair, finish your final rinse with a blast of the most freezing cold water you can bear. It closes the hair cuticles so that light bounces off them, resulting in super-shiny locks.

DON'T SKIMP ON CONDITIONER

Most hairdressers agree that healthy hair cannot be bought from a bottle, but that even if you skimp on the less expensive brands of shampoo, it is always worth investing in a good-quality conditioner. It is the equivalent of face cream for your hair.

CHECK LABELS FOR ALCOHOL

Some hair products contain alcohol which can make hair dryer than normal. If hair is coloured it tends to make it dull and less vibrant. So look carefully at the list of ingredients and avoid this ingredient.

SHINE WITH SILICA

Studies have shown that this vital mineral can stimulate healthier hair growth, and make hair stronger as well as shinier. It is found in red and green peppers, or it can be taken as a supplement.

MAKE TIME FOR MASSAGE

When you apply conditioner, give yourself a slow fingertip scalp
massage. Using gentle circular motions and a reasonable amount
of pressure pushing down onto the scalp, you will boost blood
circulation around the follicle and stimulate re-growth.

SPLASH OUT ON GOOD PRODUCTS

Many supermarket shampoos and conditioners contain very cheap
ingredients, like ammonium laurel sulfate, which are harsh on
your hair. Buy good-quality salon products and you will notice the
difference in shine and texture.

EAT NUTS FOR HEALTHY HAIR

Calcium, magnesium and potassium are all essential for the growth of
thick, healthy hair. Snack regularly on almonds that are packed with
these nutrients and contain more calcium than any other nut.

LEAVE IT LOOSE IN BED

Never jump into bed with your hair tied up in a scrunchy, or with
clips and pins still in it. Your movements throughout the course of the
night will damage and break your hair as it rubs against the pillows.

GREAT LENGTHS

Hair products containing copper peptides have already shown a
remarkable ability to increase growth. The mineral is thought to
increase thickness and reduce brittleness in hair.

SMOKING DAMAGES YOUR HAIR

Smoking is very damaging as it affects the take-up of vitamin C and
constricts the blood vessels, which means fewer of the nutrients that
are needed for hair growth are getting through. Stop smoking and you
will see instant results.

ADD MOISTURE WITH A MASK

If you feel your hair needs a pick-me-up, try an intensive conditioner or hair mask that can be left on for 10 minutes to moisturize the hair shafts. While you are waiting, wrap hair up in a warm towel to enable the treatment to penetrate more deeply.

NATURALLY STRONGER

If your hair has become weaker and more brittle with a tendency to break easily, try an infusion of rosemary poured over as a final rinse to strengthen it, or massage some rosemary essential oil (mixed with a carrier oil) onto your scalp to help promote growth and strength.

HOT HONEY HAIR

Give your hair and scalp a treat with an organic honey and olive oil conditioner. Mix equal parts together and warm in the microwave, then apply to clean, towel-dried hair, and wrap in a warm towel for 20 minutes. This will leave hair smooth and ultra-soft and shiny.

HAIR ANALYSIS EATING STRATEGY

Mineral testing a small lock of hair can reveal your metabolic type, toxin levels, health status and nutritional imbalances. Analyzing the biochemical make-up of an individual, and taking remedial action, can result in clearer skin, shinier hair, increased energy and even weight loss.

ONE HUNDRED OF THE BEST

Don't use a brush on wet hair as this could damage it. Instead use a wide-toothed comb to gently ease out knots. However, giving dry hair the traditional brushing before bedtime will benefit your locks because it stimulates growth and oil production. Natural bristle brushes are gentlest on the hair.

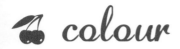 *colour*

SEAL DYE WITH VINEGAR

Rinse just-dyed hair with diluted white vinegar as a final rinse. This seals your colour so it won't fade as quickly and you can wait longer between treatments.

MIX AND MATCH

For a more unique look, mix two shades (it's a good idea to stick to the same brand) to create your own colour. Go for darker tones on the layers underneath and lighter ones at the top and front of your hair.

SINKING IN

Mist the ends of your hair with water before home-colouring. The ends of your hair are more porous and, as a result, absorb more pigment. Wet hair doesn't absorb colour as readily as dry hair. This will help you achieve an even colour while using less product.

HOME HELP

While highlights can be complicated, covering up grey hair or trying a new all-over colour is easy to do yourself. Home-dye kits are now hydrating and user-friendly. The key to dyeing your hair at home is to only go one or two shades darker or lighter, and no more.

ROOT TOUCH UP

To touch up your roots at home, start at your hairline and, using a brush applicator, brush the dye into the roots, being careful not to miss any areas. Divide the rest of your hair into sections and brush the dye into your roots section by section. Getting a friend to help will make doing the back of your head easier.

SAVVY SHAMPOOING

If you dye your hair, a great money-saving idea is to always use shampoos that are designed for colour-treated hair. You'll cut down on how frequently you need to re-dye because these shampoos are designed not to strip the colour.

NATURAL HIGHLIGHTS

Sun exposure lightens your hair naturally and you can heighten the
effects by squirting your hair with lemon juice and letting it dry in the
sun. This can be very drying for your hair, though, so follow exposure
with deep-conditioning home treatments.

RHUBARB LIGHTENER

For a natural lightening effect, simmer 4 tablespoons of powdered
rhubarb root in 700 ml (24 fl oz) of water for 30 minutes, steep for
several hours, strain, then rinse through your hair several times. Rhubarb
root can be purchased from health food stores and Chinese herbalists.

GO SEMI-NATURAL

Maintaining a bleached blonde look can be costly when your natural
colour is more mousey than Scandinavian. Try a combination of a
natural brunette shade with blonde and bronze highlights for a fair
look that's less high maintenance.

EMBRACE YOUR DARK SIDE

Many celebrities, including Madonna, Sarah Jessica Parker and
Britney Spears, have proudly shown off their dark roots. You can too
– just make sure the rest of your appearance is well groomed to avoid
looking sloppy.

STICK TO THE T

If you have fine to medium-thick hair then you can ask for a partial
T-section instead of getting a full head of highlights. The colourist
will apply highlights just on your parting and around your face. This
method is cheaper and your hair will look thicker because the darker
hair underneath the highlights creates the illusion of depth.

HOME HIGHLIGHTS

Buy a home-highlighting kit designed for your length of hair. Those
with short hair should chose one that includes a cap, while those with
long hair should pick a kit that includes an application brush that lets
you "paint" on the highlights. For best results, perform highlights on
completely dry, slightly dirty hair.

A CAP FOR BLONDES

If you have bleached or naturally blonde hair, avoid chlorine, which can make your hair turn green. Cover up with a swimming hat or use anti-chlorine shampoo to keep your colour looking natural.

HIGH OR LOWLIGHTS?

A highlight lightens and brightens the hair whereas a lowlight darkens and deepens. Highlights are blonde or gold; lowlights can be plum, auburn or chestnut, Usually two or three colours are used throughout for a multifaceted, super-shiny look. Don't go for more than that or you will scatter the strong effect.

CARROT JUICE FOR REDHEADS

If you're an orange tone redhead, enhance your natural colour with carrot juice left on the hair for five minutes and shampooed out as normal. The carrot pigment will boost the orange tones and leave your hair looking thick and colour conditioned.

COLOUR IN THE SEASONS

Get a lift of colour in the late autumn with lowlights. By this time you will have noticed that the ends of your hair are lighter in colour, but also much duller as a lasting result from summer exposure to the sun. A few highlights or lowlights will brighten the hair and act as a winter tonic to perk up your look.

BEET UP YOUR RED

For a great post-shampoo colour rinse for red-toned hair, infuse a chopped beetroot in hot water for ten minutes and use the water to rinse clean hair through to boost the natural red tones of hair and add depth and richness to colour.

BRUNETTE BOOST

Enhance the tone and shine of brunette hair by rinsing with cold coffee. Make a pot of coffee, let it cool completely, then use it as a rinse after shampooing.

GET RICH WITH ROSEMARY

To make the most of hair colour, add richness to brunette hair by infusing rosemary in hot water for ten minutes and allow to cool until warm. After shampooing, rinse through with infused water, followed by a small cold-water rinse to add shine.

COLOUR BLONDE WITH CAMOMILE

A great way to enhance shine and colour in blonde hair is to use cool camomile tea as a rinse following hair washing. This coats the hair and allows the natural blondeness to come through without product build-up.

BE KIND TO BLEACHED HAIR

If your hair is bleached, use a mild shampoo and the strongest conditioner possible without making your hair go limp, and wash your hair only as often as is necessary to avoid unnecessary drying.

CAMOUFLAGE GREY HAIRS

Older hair takes colour less well than young hair and skin. Instead of an all-over block colour, try highlights or lowlights, which give hair a sun-kissed appearance without appearing unnatural.

DO THE DIRTY

Don't turn up at the hair salon for a re-colour with freshly washed hair. Roots show up better on unwashed hair, which is also easier to handle.

BLACK IS NOT FOR BLONDES

Don't be tempted to go too dark in colour if you're naturally blonde. Dark hair tones can flatten out skin and leave you feeling dull as dishwater. If you want to go darker, do it in stages and opt for lowlights rather than all-over colour.

BE A RINSE PRINCESS

Instead of trying to dye your hair at home, which can lead to unnatural looking results, use a conditioning colour rinse, which will highlight natural colour and help boost the condition of hair as well.

NO MORE THAN FOUR

Never dye your hair more than four shades darker than its natural colour. It could wash out the colour in your eyes and skin, and leave you feeling pale and pasty.

GLOVE UP

When dying your own hair, always wear gloves to protect your hands and nails from staining, and apply a layer of moisturizer or Vaseline around the hairline to protect skin.

SUSTAIN COLOUR WITH SPF

The darker your hair colour, the more important it is to use hair products with SPF protection – sun can bleach away richness, leaving the colour flat and dull.

PASS ON THE PPDS

If you're going to dye your hair, choose natural vegetable dye rather than dyes containing PPD (Paraphenylenediamine), which can sink into skin and cause health problems. This is particularly important for dark colours, which contain higher levels.

COLOUR TO MATCH YOUR SKIN

If you have pale skin, avoid hair colours that are too light or white. Instead, go for honey blondes to enhance the natural rose tones of your skin and keep you looking healthy rather than washed out.

VEG OUT THE GREY

The best way to cover grey hair is to opt for a shade lighter than your own in a natural vegetable dye, which will colour the hair naturally without drying or causing damage.

AVOID HENNA FOR GREY HAIR

Don't use henna if you want to disguise grey hair because it won't give you a natural colour block – colour will come out redder and brighter on grey hairs, drawing attention rather than hiding them away.

COLOUR FOR VOLUME

Colour boosts volume, giving extra benefit to thin or long hair. However, your volume-boosting shampoo and conditioner may no longer be the right choice if you've coloured your hair. Experiment with different products to see what suits you.

DON'T DIY

Resorting to products from the pharmacy may end in disaster and ultimately you will have to visit a salon to put everything right, at greater expense than if you had gone there in the first place. Never correct your colour by yourself as it will only compound the problem, but visit a salon and get professional advice.

LIGHTEN UP

As skin loses melanin and becomes paler in colour, think about changing hair colour to complement your skin. Adding darker shades will drain the colour from your face, whereas a mixture of lighter shades with darker tones underneath will create texture and movement.

FRINGE BENEFITS

All types of fringes (bangs) can be flattering to older faces, but they should never look neglected with root regrowth. Most salons offer special fringe colouring services, so keep yours fully highlighted and it will lift the look of your face and the rest of your hair.

AVOID EXTREME COLOUR

Peroxide blonde and Cruella de Ville black are both very difficult shades to wear successfully as you get older. These extreme shades will draw attention to the face, and you will need superb make-up at all times to balance the effect of such dramatic hair.

KEEP IT UNDER WRAPS

Maintain colour-treated hair by keeping it from undue exposure to sunlight and chlorine. Use a bathing cap when you swim, wear hats in very sunny or poor weather and use a good-quality shampoo, formulated to help resist colour fade.

COLOUR ME BEAUTIFUL

Changing hair colour to warm up a mousy brown or cover the odd
streak of grey can take years off your age. For the most natural look
it's best to stay within two or three shades of your original colour, and
always consider your skin tone.

BEWARE SUN-IN PRODUCTS

Never use sun-lightening products, such as lemon juice or over-the-
counter products that are meant to lighten hair in the sun, or you may
soon find yourself needing a short haircut to prune away the damage.

SUNKISSED MOUSY BLONDES

As you age, skin gets paler and loses colour, so mousy hair should
be lifted with warm golden highlights to add warmth to your face.
Adding darker shades will drain even more colour from your skin.

DULL HIGHLIGHTS

In between trips to the salon, perk up dull highlights by using a
colour-enhancing treatment, or adding vitamin E oil capsules to your
weekly hair mask, to brighten colour and add shine.

COVER UP COLOUR TREATMENTS

Keep coloured hair under a scarf or broad brimmed hat when you
are out in the sunshine. UVA rays will lift the colour, and leave you
rushing to the hairdresser.

GO FOR RED

An alternative to natural highlights and lowlights is a whole head
colour change to either soft red or burnt copper, both of which are
good choices for older skin tones.

SHOP AROUND

There are so many different types of products available for every different type of hair, so make sure you find the right formula for you. Coloured hair needs a colour-formulated shampoo which will cleanse gently and won't strip the colour out.

KEEP A REGULAR TOUCH UP

Nothing is more ageing than large grey roots on coloured hair. In order to avoid this you will have to make sure you book an appointment at least every six weeks.

CHECK OUT YOUR BROWS

Often the colour of the brows fades as you get older and you will need to assess your hair colour in combination with your brows. If you don't, you run the change of having a beautiful head of hair that is detracted by pale or greying brows. Get the objective professional advice of a colourist before making a decision.

CUT DOWN ON CHEMICALS

Professional hairdressers suggest that in order to keep hair as healthy as it can be, you choose only one chemical treatment at a time. For example, perming and colouring together will leave hair weak, chemically damaged and very brittle.

HOLIDAY HAIRCARE

Always wash your hair as soon as possible after swimming in the sea or a chlorinated swimming pool. Coloured and treated hair are prone to damage and fading if sea salt or chemicals are left in the hair, especially if you intend to spend time out in the sun after your swim.

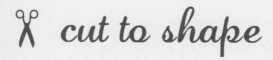

cut to shape

SEE AN EXPERT
The number one tip for great hair is to get a good haircut. They can be expensive, but you're likely to recoup all the money you've spent on a quality professional because you'll need far fewer products (and time) to make it look good once you get home. The style will keep its shape for longer, too.

SQUARE UP TO SOFT LAYERS
If you have a square-shaped face, steer clear of bobs or short styles that accentuate your strong jawline. Instead, go for softer layers around the face to break up and cut into the squareness, and bring more attention to eyes and forehead.

LAYER IT OVAL
Oval faces are the most versatile face shape for styles. They do, however, work best with layers, long or short, which enhance the natural bone structure without lengthening the chin and dragging down the face. Oval faces should avoid blunt fringes and harsh crops.

SQUARE THE CIRCLE
Round-faced people should avoid fringes and styles that are cropped close or pulled back on the sides of the face. All round fullness is best and crops work well because of the added volume around the face.

LAYER IT FULL
Having your hair cut with layers all over, rather than just at the front, will increase the appearance of fullness, making it look larger than life without the need for over-styling.

CHOOSE CAREFULLY
Choose your hairdresser carefully. High-street haircuts can be quite limiting because many chains have specific styles for each season and diversification is discouraged. Make sure your hairdresser is working to make you look your best.

HEART YOUR FRINGE

Heart-shaped faces are perfect for fringes – it will slim down the forehead and accentuate the bones of the lower face. Height on top of the head also works, but beware of long, straight hair or centre partings that can drag the face down.

AVOID THE TRIANGLE

If you are growing out hair from a mid to a longer length, you may find that the weight of the hair makes the crown look skull-tight and the ends appear thicker – creating a horrid triangle shape from crown to shoulders. This is flattering to no one, so make sure you get the shape re-cut as it grows to accommodate a style suitable for longer hair.

GIVE FINE HAIR THE CHOP

Very fine hair should not be grown past the shoulders as it will look thin and weak – if it is blonde it may even seem transparent. Layers and blunt cuts work well, but pay attention to strengthening the hair on the sides of the face where hair is weakest – a fringe may help remedy the problem.

GET FRINGE BENEFITS

If you want a change of style without having lots chopped off, ask for a fringe. It will transform your look dramatically. Feathery styles are kinder and easier to maintain than the severe Cleopatra look.

BE BLUNT

If your hair is thinning or looking fine and wispy, go for blunt ended haircuts rather than feathering. Blunt ends give hair the appearance of being thicker.

DON'T GO TOO LONG

Very long hair, way down your back, can look far too teenage once you are past 35; in fact, it can make you look a lot older than you are. If you love your long hair and don't want to give it up, try trimming off just 5 cm (2 inches) and seeing what it looks like. If you like it, get a little more trimmed off. You may find your face becomes the focal point rather than your hair, with a prettier result!

GO SHORTER

Ageing skin and faces ordinarily look better with lighter, shorter
haircuts. This is because long hair can "drag" the face down, making
wrinkles appear worse. Also, the shorter your haircut, the more
volume it will appear to have.

GET THE BEST FROM YOUR STYLIST

Book a quiet appointment time, like first thing on a Monday morning.
When the salon is quiet, your hairdresser will have more time to focus
on you, and give you exactly what you want.

READ A MAGAZINE

Take a look at some of the hair magazines on offer, as they will be
showing the season's latest styles, cuts and colours. Even if they seem
a little young or trendy to you, there are often ways of adapting them
that can keep you in fashion but also within your comfort zone.

CALL A FRIEND

Ask a friend or family member for their realistic opinion but be
prepared that they might not be flattering. An honest opinion delivered
by someone who knows you can really put you in touch with what's not
working for you. Remember that they are probably more used to your
face and the way it looks in various situations than you are.

ALL CHANGE

It's important to keep "tweaking" your hairstyle, and not to become
trapped in a style that suited you when you were a teenager.
Sometimes the best way to change your style, is to try a new stylist or
go to a salon that has a different approach than your usual one. All it
takes is for someone to see you in a slightly new way.

DON'T GO TOO SHORT

Unless you have an amazingly elfin face, short cropped hair can look
very butch and severe. Try a short bob instead, which is sleek and
sophisticated and suits a greater variety of face shapes.

INDULGE IN A LITTLE CHIT-CHAT

Always find time for a five-minute chat with your hairdresser to discuss exactly what you want. This time is vital for them to look at the texture of your hair and your face shape before they start to work on you. If you've been with them for a while, they will also be able to pick up on changes that you might not have noticed – such as a few more grey hairs, thinning, or poor condition or split ends – and find remedies for them.

FLATTERING CUTS

Make your haircut work for you. Choose a hairstyle that has a side fringe (bangs) rather than a straight-across fringe, and a length that falls to just below the chin if you want to cover a wrinkled forehead and sagging jaw.

THE PERFECT LENGTH

The most flattering and youthful hair length, post 40, is to just below the chin to cover the jawline. This length works on nearly all women and the hair can swing above the shoulder.

HEAVY HAIR SHADOWS SKIN

A thick and solid curtain of glossy hair can overwhelm the face and make skin look dull and tired. Shorter layers, cut through from underneath, are needed to give movement around the face and let light shine through.

A LONG BOB

If your hair is in good condition and you are prepared to spend time blow-drying, a long bob is a good option, as the hair swings to create movement and will cover a jowly jawline and wrinkled neck.

AN UNFORGIVING CUT

Cropped hair can look fabulous on older women, but avoid a close-cut crop if you are bigger than a size 14 (US size 10), as visually it does not balance a larger frame.

WITH A FRINGE ON TOP

A badly wrinkled forehead is easy to cover up with a fringe (bangs). Depending on your face shape, your fringe can be straight and solid or soft and wispy, but it will do the trick of hiding frown lines.

KEEP HAIR SOFT

Blunt geometric bobs that need a blast of hairspray to keep them in place can look hard and severe as the face ages and loses its youthful bloom. A good haircut for an older woman needs to have movement and softness around the face.

CUTS THAT FLATTER

Try to avoid layered short cuts, as they can be very ageing by exposing a saggy, wrinkled neck. If you have your hair a little longer, consider just feathering the fringe (bangs) and sides which will keep the look soft and flattering.

healthy hair

PROTECT AGAINST HEAT DAMAGE

Use a thermal protection product before you blow-dry or straighten your hair, especially if you have very curly or Afro-style hair. The conditioners and polymers in the products will protect your hair.

THICKEN HAIR WITH MASSAGE

One of the signs of ageing is thinning hair. We all lose between 50–100 strands of hair every day but if you're losing more, get a head massage – it will stimulate the roots and help hair growth.

POMEGRANATE POWER

Pomegranate oil is a salon-standard hot-oil treatment. Simply heat in warm water and apply to your hair before shampooing to soothe and condition. Pomegranate oil will enhance the appearance and feel of your hair, help with detangling and moisturize the hair shaft.

DO THE TWIST AND SNIP

One temporary method for removing split ends, though not a solution, is to twist a small strand of hair gently until the damaged and split ends appear, sticking out. Holding a pair of scissors vertically, carefully snip off these ends. You will only be trimming the split ends, not the length.

PREVENT BROKEN SHAFTS

Damage to hair, often caused by rough mishandling and using elastic bands that break the hair mid-shaft, can be prevented by taking better care. Do not brush your hair when it's wet, use soft fabric bands or scrunchies to hold your hair back and avoid robust towel drying – instead wrap your hair in a towel and pat and squeeze gently to absorb excess water.

PRE-SHAMPOO BOOSTER

There's no need to spend a fortune on the pre-shampoo treatments that hairstylists try to sell you these days. Brushing your dry hair thoroughly before showering should remove product build-up and help stimulate the scalp to promote blood flow, which in turn delivers strengthening nutrients to hair follicles.

END SPLIT ENDS

Split ends are the bane of anyone with medium to long hair, but they can be prevented by getting regular six-week trims. For an existing problem, use a product formulated for repairing ends. These are applied to the tips of the hair and left in – they won't mend the hair but they will minimize the "split" appearance. Fortify the hair by using a strengthening shampoo and conditioner.

DAMAGE LIMITATION

Rather than diet or environment, it is usually mistreatment that causes hair damage. Bleaching, perming, chemical straightening and the overuse of hot appliances all break down the outer cuticle of the hair. The more you indulge in these techniques, the more damaged your hair will be, so limit your exposure. For example, if you lighten your hair, avoid daily use of a blow-dryer or straightener – you can't have it all.

DETOX DULL HAIR

Use a clarifying shampoo once a week to remove build-up of styling products and accumulated conditioner. Product residue weighs down hair, makes it difficult to style and dulls colour.

POST-40 HAIR

A sad fact is that after 40, and especially during the menopause, hair thins in diameter and hair growth slows, so we produce less hairs. You may find that changing your haircare regime to avoid harsh products and styling may help redress the problem.

AFRO DOES IT

Only use hair products specially formulated for Afro hair – these will not overstrip the hair and will keep the cuticles conditioned and soft. Products with EFA (essential fatty acids) that resemble the natural sebum of the hair will nourish both scalp and hair.

GROW STRONG AND LONG

Although hair grows only 15 cm (6 in) a year, and you are unlikely to greatly increase this rate, B vitamins, betacarotene and a protein-rich diet may help maximize your growth cycle. Keep your hair one length and always comb from the bottom up, section by section, to avoid breakages.

SCOFF SALMON FOR SHINY TRESSES

Salmon is the number one food for shiny, glossy hair. The fish oils it contains plump up the cuticle and keep hair moisturized without being greasy. Other oily fish are good, too – try sardines, anchovies and mackerel.

FIX THE FUZZ

Short hairs around the parting and forehead are a sign of damaged new hair growth. Stress or poor nutrition may be to blame, but this could also be a result of directing a blow-dryer at the roots of your hair. To remedy, use a strengthening serum, don't blow-dry near the area and have a deep conditioning treatment in a salon. In the meantime, smooth the fuzzy hairs with a conditioning styling cream, not a serum.

FLAKE BE GONE

Instead of sticking to an anti-dandruff shampoo all the time, which can be drying, try alternating it with another type of shampoo, so you can help keep your hair in good condition and your dandruff at bay.

DON'T FLAKE OUT

If you suffer from recurrent dandruff or an itchy scalp, try treating your head with tea tree oil, which has been shown to reduce dandruff by up to 40% in sufferers.

EAT AWAY HAIR LOSS

Hair loss happens at times of stress and anxiety, often when diet degenerates. Stick to healthy foods like fruit and vegetables to give hair a boost and breathe deeply to replenish oxygen levels.

KELP IT THICK

Sea kelp supplements are thought to help thicken hair with their marine ingredients, which not only promote hair growth and prevent sun and pollution damage, but also add essential micronutrients to the hair root.

TIE ON A TURBAN

Instead of rubbing hair with a towel, pat it dry instead – wet hair is extremely fragile and rubbing can cause damage to hair shafts. The best way is to wrap hair loosely in a dry towel directly after shampooing to allow the cotton towel to naturally absorb the water. Do not put it on top of the head, which can stretch and knot hair strands, but wrap it along the length, just as it is done in the hair salon.

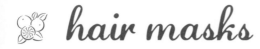 # hair masks

THICKEN UP WITH WHEAT
To give yourself thick, glossy, catwalk hair and restore flexibility, strength and shine, apply a wheatgerm mask. Soak a little wheatgerm, which is rich in vitamin E, in hot water for five minutes, then drain it and apply the residue to the hair. Leave for five minutes, then rinse hair thoroughly.

MOISTURIZE WITH OLIVE OIL
Olive oil is nature's great moisturizer. Give yourself a deep-conditioning hot oil hair wrap by massaging gently warmed olive oil into the hair and scalp, then wrap your head in a warm towel (which has been heated in a tumble dryer briefly) for 10–20 minutes. Follow by shampooing, conditioning and drying as usual.

COCONUT SHINE
Coconut has long been known for its moisturizing effects. Make your own hair treat by combining coconut oil with a teaspoon of honey for a ten-minute boosting mask that will rescue dry or damaged hair. Those with very dry or curly hair may benefit from massaging the coconut oil into the hair and leaving it on overnight as it naturally softens, conditions and relaxes the hair.

KEEP YOUR HAIR ON
Tea leaves and lemon juice can be used to prevent hair loss and also help you enhance the natural shine of your hair. Boil and strain tea, then add lemon juice as it cools and use as a conditioner before rinsing thoroughly.

GET FRUITY FOR EXTRA SHINE
Control oily build-up and add shine with a fruity hair rinse. Heat a sliced orange, a sliced apple and a small slice of melon with 1 litre (2 pints) of water in a saucepan for ten minutes. Strain and allow to cool, then add 500 ml (1 pint) of cider vinegar. Leave for 24 hours before using to rinse hair.

LEAVE IN A HONEY SHINE

For a leave-in treatment that gives extra shine, dissolve a teaspoon of honey into 500 ml (1 pint) of warm water. After shampooing, pour the mixture through the hair, distributing evenly. Do not rinse out, and dry as normal.

LIGHTEN UP WITH LEMON

Lemon juice and vinegar are both excellent for oily hair. They will also give lustre to blonde hair and bring out highlights. Never pour vinegar or lemon juice directly onto your hair; dilute them first with water and distribute evenly.

GIVE YOUR SHAMPOO AN ADDITIVE

Boil a couple of handfuls of mint leaves in 1 litre (2 pints) of water for 20 minutes. Strain and add the mint infusion into a bottle of normal shampoo. Because mint is clarifying, detoxing and cleansing, the infusion is best suited to those with oily-to-normal hair.

TONE YOUR SCALP

Mix a tablespoon of malt vinegar in a glass of water, and add a pinch of salt. Massage into your scalp with the fingertips and repeat twice a week, leaving on for an hour before rinsing in cold water. The vinegar solution will cleanse and tone the scalp, prevent oiliness and add shine to the hair.

DIY SHAMPOO MASK

Whisk together equal amounts of castor oil, glycerine, cider vinegar and a mild herbal shampoo. Massage into the hair like a normal shampoo, but leave on for 10–20 minutes before rinsing. The shampoo mask will add shine to dull, lacklustre hair.

SHINE UP AN EGG

For flyaway hair, make a homemade conditioning mask to reduce static and add shine by whisking an egg with 200 g (7 oz) of natural (plain) yogurt and massaging into the scalp. Leave for a few minutes, then rinse thoroughly.

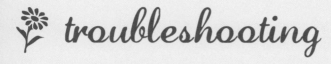 *troubleshooting*

TEA TREATMENT
Greasy hair will benefit from a weekly treatment of cold peppermint tea, poured over the hair after washing. It will also make your hair smell fresh and minty for 24 hours.

STRESS-RELATED DANDRUFF
Internal stress and conflict trigger many physical signs that your life is unbalanced. When the glands that produce oil start overworking, dead cells fall off in clumps rather than one by one, and cause dandruff. Try using a shampoo containing zinc, sulphur or selenium.

FLAKY WHITE DANDRUFF
The shiny white scales that separate from the scalp and collect on the hair and shoulders are almost always caused by an impaired general health. Increase your intake of raw foods that are high in enzymes (fruit, vegetables and nuts) and take two dessertspoons of flax oil a day until the condition improves.

MOISTURIZE YOUR SCALP
A flaky scalp can be a sign of dryness and a result of poor diet, stress or fluctuating hormones. It should be treated with products that add moisture like aloe-vera shampoo and conditioner.

REPAIR CENTRAL-HEATING DAMAGE
The contrast of chilly outdoor temperatures and warm central heating can cause a dry, itchy scalp. Look for a mild shampoo from an organic range, which will be kind to your hair and will provide it with plant-based extractions to soothe the scalp.

SPIRIT CLEANSING

Any kind of alcoholic drink will have a drying effect when applied to oily hair. The higher the alcohol content, the better the effect. Mix a shot glass of vodka, or whatever spirit you have, with a couple of cups of water and rinse through your hair.

BE AN EGGHEAD

Run out of shampoo? Beat two eggs in a cup of warm water. Add a squirt of lemon juice if you have oily hair. Massage the mixture through your hair, leave on for ten minutes then rinse with warm water. Make sure the water isn't too hot or you'll end up with scrambled egg on your head!

COLOUR CODING

Turn no-frills shampoo into a bespoke product. Add a cooled cup of camomile tea to enhance blonde hair and boiled and strained rosemary leaves for brunettes.

SHAMPOO STRETCHER

If you can't give up your favourite expensive shampoo, make it last longer. Put a bit of bicarbonate of soda (baking soda) in your hand with a small blob of shampoo, then lather up for more froth with less product.

EMERGENCY HAND CREAM FOR HAIR

In an emergency you can use a tiny amount of light hand cream to control frizzy hair without damaging it. Rub a small amount of cream into your hands, and when it is almost absorbed run your hands very lightly down the length of your hair; make sure you give your hair a deep conditioning treatment the next day.

KITCHEN COLOUR CORRECTOR

If blonde hair turns a strange shade of "green" after a summer spent swimming in chlorinated pools, comb tomato ketchup through and leave for 20 minutes to neutralize colour. Afterwards wash and condition in the usual way.

SUNLIGHT STEALS MOISTURE

A summer vacation will leave your hair feeling dry and brittle, as the UV rays suck out moisture. Every other day apply a leave-in conditioner that has a UV filter for protection.

SUNSHINE INCREASES THE GREASE

Hot summer sunshine can increase sweat production and make your scalp look and feel much greasier. To counteract this problem, try more frequent washing with a small amount of shampoo, and use a much lighter conditioner.

DETOX POLLUTED HAIR

In the summer months there are higher levels of humidity and pollution in the air, so hair should be washed and conditioned more frequently. Use a good detox shampoo, which will clean the hair gently without stripping away natural oils.

SUNLIGHT DAMAGES PRODUCTS

Keep conditioners and styling products away from the beach, as they need to be kept in a cool, shady place. Exposure to strong sunlight will destroy some of the active ingredients that make these hair products work.

REMEDY SCARECROW HAIR

A week of sun, salt water, and chlorine will all play havoc with your hair, so spend one beach day with your hair covered in an intensive conditioner, slicked back, and covered with a fashionable Pucci- or Hermes-style scarf. This eight-hour treatment will restore your hair to pre-vacation condition.

WIND WARNING

Strong winds can cause almost as much damage as the sun to your hair in summer, so occasionally use a good leave-in conditioner that contains Vitamin B5, which will nourish and protect your hair from damage. Wear a hat if you are going to be out in extreme weather conditions.

EXTEND YOUR LOCKS

As age takes its toll on the speed of hair growth, you can always cheat a little with some longer extensions. The process is lengthy and extensions need to be put in professionally, but they can add volume and length very successfully. If your hair is very thin, keep them at shoulder-length or above.

KNOW THIN FROM FINE

Thin hair and fine hair are different and need to be treated differently. Thin or "low density" hair has a less-than-average number of strands per square centimetre, so that the scalp can sometimes be seen through the hair. This can be in patches or all over. Fine hair – of which you can have in abundance – refers to the thickness of the strands and can resemble thin hair because both types tend to be flat and lie close to the head.

PREVENTION IS THE BEST CURE

Breakages and poor condition are some of the reasons hair thins, so take steps to prevent hair loss by restricting the use of blow-dryers – extreme heat can break down the proteins in hair – straighteners or chemical treatments such as perms, straightening agents and colouring. The more you abuse your hair, the more risk there is of long-term damage.

ADD VOLUME WITH LAYERS

Choose a style that falls above the shoulder line, and that has layers cut into it for extra volume. Always use volumizing shampoos and styling products. A little mousse can be used to pump up the layers, but be careful not to overload the hair with product.

CLEVER COVER-UP

If you find your hair thinning at your parting line, pull the front section of hair up over the top of your head and secure with a clip at the crown, to cover up the parting.

USE VOLUMIZING SHAMPOO SPARINGLY

Avoid using a specially formulated volumizing shampoo all the time, because the proteins they use to bond with the hair can build up as a residue and make hair look dull and lifeless.

COLOUR-CORRECT THIN HAIR

Avoid all-over flat colour and instead try several shades of high and lowlights. These add body and contrast to the hair, creating the illusion of depth.

SEAWEED REMEDY

To improve the thickness and condition of your hair take a daily sea kelp supplement. This broad-fronded seaweed comes in several varieties but all are rich in the minerals potassium, calcium, magnesium and iron.

VOLUMIZE THIN HAIR

After washing your hair, apply a thickening spray and blow-dry through, using your fingers to create a messy, tousled look. This look works best on mid-length layered cuts.

THIN ON TOP

Hair naturally thins out as part of the ageing process, as the number of follicles capable of growing hairs gradually declines. A straight parting with hair that just hangs down from it will emphasize this problem, so ask your stylist to create a style for you that incorporates colour and texture.

THIN HAIR SOLUTIONS

If you find your hair losing body as well as volume as you age, you need to find a style that incorporates some layering, whatever the length. Keeping hair cut all the same length can drag it down and make it look even thinner.

FINE-HAIR FULLNESS

Traditional layers do not work as well for fine hair unless they are simple bevelled edges; instead try a perm which thickens the diameter of the strands. This can be done on large rollers for waves rather than the classic kinky perm you might remember from your youth.

GUARD AGAINST HAIR LOSS

Thinning hair that falls out in clumps can come about as a result of a restricted diet. Hair loss from lack of vitamins B, C and iron can be rectified with a diet rich in protein and vegetables. Packed with EFAs (essential fatty acids), flax seeds will make hair thicker and shinier.

AVOID TIGHT STYLES

Tight ponytails or cornrows can put stress on hair and also increase the chance of breakages and hair loss. Frequently winding the hair around rollers, particularly the non-foam varieties, can also worsen hair loss.

GET WIGGY WITH IT

If ageing has caused your hair to thin down so much that you can see your scalp through it, then a good-quality wig is an option. You can get it cut and thinned down to the right weight for you by a professional hairdresser.

going grey

GREY HEADS GO BLONDE

Occasionally grey hair can acquire a yellow tint; this can be avoided by choosing shampoos and conditioners that have been specially formulated for highlighted hair.

FADE TO GREY

When our bodies stop producing the pigment melanin our hair starts to turn grey. This won't happen overnight, but having highlights around the crown will soothe the transition to a full head of grey hair, and will help create warmth and depth to the salt-and-pepper colour, whatever your style.

GREY MATTERS

By the age of 50, 50% of women will be 50% grey. Grey hair doesn't have to mean "old" hair. No matter what the shade, hair is an extension of who we are, and if it is glossy, well cared for and cut regularly, you will look fabulous whatever your colour.

A BRAND NEW SHADE

If you find yourself with too much grey hair and want to turn back the clock to how it used to look, never go for the exact same shade; try one shade lighter as it will be more flattering to your skin tone.

THE HIGHS AND LOWS

As the number of grey flecks in your hair start to increase, highlighted hair becomes less flattering. Try asking for highlights and lowlights at the same time to complement your new salt-and-pepper growth.

HAIR LOSS MAKES GREY MORE OBVIOUS

Drug treatments for illnesses, even if they are alternative medicine, can arrest the growth cycle of hair and cause it to fall out, as can alopecia, a condition that causes hair loss. When hair is lost, more of the existing greys may be revealed.

FIRST GREY HAIRS

At the beginning of the greying process, usually around your late thirties, follicles produce colourless strands in a random pattern, often on the temples and the top of your head. Darker hairs normally hide the grey strands when they first appear. At this stage it is unlikely that anyone other than you will notice the grey. If you are worried, changing your parting may make those strands a little less noticeable

WHITEN THE GREY

Technically there is no such hair colour as grey. Hair is either pigmented or it is white – the grey is simply a mixture of white hair and coloured hair. If your grey hair looks dull, consider using a silver shampoo formula, which will brighten both the white and pigmented strands and give them lustre.

FEED YOUR HAIR

Because hair grows with the melanin pigment inside, no external cause will make you go grey. To keep melanin production at a high level, ensure you are getting enough of the mineral copper in your diet. Food that contains good supplies include crab, oysters, sunflower seeds and nuts.

WHEN TO COVER THE GREY

If your hair is just beginning to change colour, with the grey making up less than 20%, use a semi-permanent colour that will begin to fade in about 6–12 washes; for up to 50% grey, opt for semi-permanent that will last for about 24 washes. Only choose a permanent dye if the majority of your hair has turned grey. If you're mostly grey, consider a shade slightly darker than your normal colour as the colour may fade with exposure to sun and shampooing.

RESTRICT YOUR DIET

To prevent premature greying some nutritionists recommend restricting your intake of caffeine, alcohol, meat and any food that is fried, greasy, spicy, sour or acidic. These items are said to reduce moisture and nutrients from reaching the hair follicles.

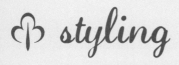 *styling*

BETTER BRUSHSTROKES

You only really need two types of brush to style your tresses: a natural-bristled round or flat brush to use on dry hair and a soft, rubber, wide-toothed comb to use on damp hair, as it stretches and snaps more easily. Brushes are inexpensive and it's worth shopping around as the right bristles will really help your hair appear smoother.

SELECT SILICONE

A drop of silicone serum will temporarily coat and smooth the hair cuticle and add shine if your hair is frizzy, dry or damaged. Use only a tiny amount to prevent any build-up and concentrate it on the ends if you have fine or greasy hair.

STAY SMOOTH AND DRY

To dry hair super-straight, use a straightening cream or serum on damp hair. Work down the hair shaft using a hairdryer with a nozzle. If your hair is prone to frizziness, don't dry it upside down or point the airflow upwards, which can roughen up the cuticle – instead, point it down the hair shaft from roots to ends.

BLOW-DRY LIKE A PRO

For super-sleek hair, use a round radial brush and blow-dryer on damp hair. Comb through a serum or thermal protector, then divide your hair into small, 5 cm (2 in) sections. Work section by section from the nape of the neck to the crown. Place the brush underneath the hair and, directing the nozzle of the hairdryer from the roots to the ends, dry along the length. Move the hairdryer constantly. Be careful not to wrap a big section of hair around the brush, otherwise you could get into a tangly mess. Finish each section with a blast of cold air.

FORESTALL THE FRIZZ

If you suffer from frizzy hair, dry hair completely before leaving the house. Kinking or frizzing can occur if hair is even just a tiny bit damp when you go out in the wind and air.

FIGHT THE FRIZZ

If your hair is curly or very prone to frizz, especially in damp weather, try to use a wide-toothed comb, which separates the hairs, rather than a brush. Avoid handling the hair too much and apply serum or a leave-in conditioner with the fingers, smoothing the hair into manageable locks or large ringlets.

KEEP KINKS AWAY

To avoid telltale kinks in long hair, do not put it in a ponytail or bun while it's wet or damp, or for at least six hours after styling if you've used styling products.

FRENCH PLAIT

For a great way to create waves, especially on thick hair, get a friend to give you a French plait while hair is still damp, then leave it in for several hours and use fingers to tease out the curls.

DON'T HEAT EXTENSIONS

If you want to style or curl acrylic hair extensions, be sure to use rollers with no thermal styling products and take care using hot blow-dryers or other styling tools. Most extensions are not made of real hair and may burn. To prolong the life of your extensions, whether they are natural or acrylic, never sleep with wet hair and do not try to dye them yourself at home – always visit a salon for colour.

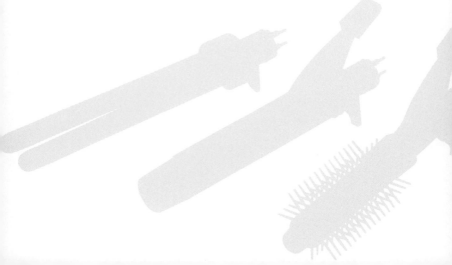

MILK THOSE STRAIGHTENERS

According to Indian tradition, milk is an excellent hair straightener. For super-straight hair, spritz milk onto the hair while it's still damp, then let it set for 20 minutes before rinsing and shampooing as usual.

ROUGH DRY HAIR BEFORE STYLING

Blow-drying isn't all bad for your hair - instead of blow-drying your hair from wet, rough dry hair until it is 80% dry, then blow-dry or style in sections to avoid heat damage.

VOLUME LIFTER

If you have long hair that can drag down with gravity, or if you have limp hair that needs extra volume, apply some volumizer spray to the roots of damp hair and add lift by blow-drying your hair upside-down. Bend over at the waist and blow-dry from the roots. Dry first at the nape of the neck and finish with the top, front layer.

STOP THE STATIC

To remedy flyaway, static hair, which can be a particular problem in hot, dry weather, spray hairspray on your brush and brush through your hair. Alternatively spritz with water, and always use a moisturizing shampoo.

VOLUMIZE WHILE WET

The most effective way to use volumizing mousse is to apply it to damp hair and then blow it dry – this will help boost body, especially if you concentrate on lifting at the roots. Use a volumizing shampoo and conditioner; a short style with lots of layers will help lift flat, lank hair.

START AT THE BACK

Apply styling products first to the back of the hair, where you have most hair, working your way forwards to the front sections. This will ensure even distribution and prevent you from adding too much product to the top of the head.

LOOK AT THE OVERALL PICTURE

Some women look great with trendy, spiky, shorter and can wear
them into their seventies with great aplomb, whereas others in their
twenties wouldn't be able to carry the look off. The key is to consider
not only the quality and texture of your hair but also your bone
structure, as well as your build, personality and dress sense – for a
look to work well all these factors need to be in tune.

NOZZLE AWAY FRIZZ

A great way to prevent frizz and flyaway hairs when blow-drying is
to use the nozzle attachment of your hairdryer, which will target hair
exactly and enable you to dry it in sections without causing other
areas to frizz up.

ROUND IT OUT

For shorter, layered styles, apply mousse and then use a round brush
to dry and style the hair. This will add volume and sleekness without
curl. Once dry, shape the style with your fingers and finish off the
ends with a little wax or gel for added definition.

GET SILKY SHINE

Smooth silk can boost the natural shine of your hair and help smooth
down follicles. Wrap a silk scarf around your hairbrush and "brush"
your hair with it to add a lustrous shine

SOFT FOAM CURLS

Avoid the heat damage of hot rollers by using bendy foam curlers to
achieve a smooth ringlet look. Apply a little setting lotion, then wind
your hair around the curlers. Leave in overnight and you will have
curls you can finger through and break up for a casual look.

SAY ALOE TO SMOOTH HAIR

If you have curly hair and don't want it to frizz, but would like to
keep that natural shine, apply a small amount of aloe vera, which will
smooth the hair shaft without weighing it down.

TRY TOUSLED TRESSES

Instead of leaving hair looking groomed to within an inch of its life, try spraying a mist of volumizing lotion onto it and style with fingers only to add texture and avoid that over-brushed look.

DRY NATURALLY

Allow hair to dry naturally as often as possible to restore hair health, rather than always reaching for the hairdryer and styling tools. If you hate your frizzy curls, apply a serum and twist large ringlets around your fingers as your hair air-dries – this creates large sleek curls rather than frizzy ones.

GET SET TO SHOWER

When using non-heated rollers, put your hair in them before taking a shower and the steam will help set the curls for a longlasting style when you take them out. Make sure you wait until the hair is fully dry before removing the rollers.

SWEET-SMELLING HAIR

Before you go out, spritz fragrance through your hair. It is more porous than skin, so you will retain the sweet-smelling aroma for longer.

CHOOSE VELCRO FOR FINE HAIR

Velcro rollers provide soft curl and full body, and can be used on either damp or dry hair. They are good choices for short or fine hair and hair that breaks easily, since they don't need to be clipped in place.

NEW DAY, NEW LOOK

For a new look without a cut, simply change your parting. If you are used to a side parting, a centre one can really make your features stand out and give you a fresher, younger look.

SHINE ON THE SPRAY

To get instant lustrous shine all over, use a spray gloss in the same way as you would hairspray. This is a gloss product that delivers a fine, light mist without leaving the heavy slickness of a serum.

SIMPLE AND STYLISH

A style that incorporates lots of hair clips or decorations are best
reserved for the under-30s. Zany, oddball or cute isn't the look to
cultivate – instead think sexy, stylish and chic. Erring on the side
of simplicity, with a great cut and colour, will make heads turn for
all the right reasons.

WAX IT UP

Wax is a great product to add shine and separation to short or medium
choppy styles. First, rub wax between the hands to warm it and then
distribute it evenly and lightly all over the hair. Do not apply it in pieces
to bits here and there as you won't get the full shine benefits.

GO LOOSE FOR ROLLERS

Never wind rollers too tightly, or you could end up with hair loss
and damage as the hair is stretched, torn or pulled out from the root.
Remember, hair contracts when drying, so if you're putting them on
wet hair, give yourself a bit of extra room.

OVER-BRUSHING CAN BE DAMAGING

Always use a good-quality brush to style your hair but do not over-
brush it, as with every stroke you will damage your hair more and
create more split ends.

LAY OFF THE HEAT

Long-term use of heated appliances will damage your hair by drying
out the shaft. If you avoid using heated products every day of the
week and save them for special occasions, you will start to notice
the improvement in the texture of your hair within weeks.

MAKE A BIG IMPRESSION

Root-lift without a salon blow-dry can be achieved by a quick
10-minute upside down root blast with a professional high-watt
hairdryer. There's no need to wash your hair first as it works
better on slightly dirty hair, and gives hair immediate lift and body.

AVOID CUTESY ACCESSORIES

Pigtails and bunches are best left to 10-year-olds. Plastic bobbles, floral clips and glitter scrunchies will all only serve to emphasize your lack of youthfulness.

BACKCOMB TO BUILD UP

If your hair has lost some of its natural body, a quick way to add volume without blow-drying is to backcomb very gently with a wide-toothed comb, and then spray with a light-formula superfine setting mist.

BE LONGLASTING WITH GEL

Suitable for short, layered or intricate styles that need firm hold, gel will allow you to shape the hair to some extent, keeping it in position. It is best applied either wet and allowed to dry naturally in shape, or after a blow-dry. If you apply it before you blow-dry, you are likely to get an unattractive flaky residue.

PICK AND CHOOSE PRODUCTS

Choose the right products for your hair type, which will change throughout your life depending on environmental factors, stress and dietary changes. If you have oily roots and dry ends, find a shampoo for oily hair and concentrate on lathering at the roots: the rest of your hair will still get clean.

LET YOUR HAIR DOWN

If you have a slack jawline, avoid putting your hair up in buns or chignons. No matter how sleek-looking, these are looks that are best suited for those with perfect profiles. Such styles can also make a thin face look even thinner —having some volume around the chin creates a more youthful fullness and hides the jawline at the same time.

CHECK OUT STYLING PRODUCTS

Hair changes as you get older, and you may need to consider products you have never used before. These can add volume, give root-lift, add gloss, help control static and protect the shaft from heated styling appliances. Check them out to make the most of your hair.

BAD HAIR DAYS

Studies at Yale University show that "bad hair days" really can effect self-esteem, increase self-doubt and intensify insecurities. Women perceive their capabilities to be significantly lower when their hair doesn't look good, so time spent with the dryer is time well spent.

BLOT UP EXCESS MOISTURE

Between showering and drying your hair, always blot hair dry with a fresh towel to absorb excess water. If you then apply a heat-activated product that coats and protects the hair shaft, you will minimize damage from the hairdryer and keep your hair in optimum condition.

STYLE IT QUICKLY

After showering wrap hair gently in a towel, choose and apply the correct amount of styling product and then blow-dry. Damp hair that is moisture-laden will help styling products work better, and you will achieve better results.

WEAR A HAT

If your roots are showing a little too much or your hair is lifeless and flat – or you simply haven't had time to look after it properly – solve the problem by donning a stylish hat. If you hate hats, try a stylish scarf or hair band to keep your locks under control.

EXTRA SHINE

If you want to make straight hair even glossier, blow-dry in the usual way and then brush through for 5 minutes from root to tip with a paddled shaped hairbrush with good-quality bristles.

POWER DRY

For a professional finish at home, look for a good-quality dryer that has between 1200 and 2000 watts. When you use it, keep the heat setting on low and the drier moving around so that heat damage is kept to a minimum.

SALON SMOOTHIE

For salon-styled hair always divide your hair into manageable sections. The more you do, the better the result. Point the hairdryer downwards to close hair shafts, making hair look ultra-sleek.

EXPERIMENT AT HOME

Even something as simple as changing your parting line can make you look younger. Take a pile of magazine cuttings, a comb and some clips, and experiment in front of the mirror to try out different styles.

BAND AID

Tying a tight black hairband up over the forehead will keep your hair sleek and tidy and help keep wrinkles pulled back. Backcomb hair slightly and let it fall down over the band like a sexy 1950s film star.

PONYTAIL PULL-UP

Try wearing your hair up in a high, sleek ponytail. It pulls the skin up towards the crown, making it appear taut and smooth, and looks tidy and chic.

styling tools

DON'T NEGLECT BRUSHES

Just like your hair, your brushes, combs and styling tools need regular washing to maintain tiptop form. Use shampoo or mild detergent to keep them sparkling clean.

PLACE YOUR ORDER

For medium-length to long hair, you're best off using a chunky, barrelled brush but often these aren't available in shops. Ask your hair stylist to order you one for a professional approach at home.

GET DRY QUICK

Brushes with holes in the base or around the barrel help the flow of air through the brush and can enable you to dry hair more quickly, boosting volume by targeting all areas of the hair shaft and root.

GO WIDE FOR THICK HAIR

Wide-spaced and staggered rows of bristles enable a brush to slip through the hair more easily, which is an important feature if you have thick, wavy or curly hair that tangles easily.

DON'T KEEP DAMAGED GOODS

When the bristles of your hairbrush start looking damaged, bent or frayed, or the brush starts losing bristles, it's time to replace your hairbrush. Over-used bristles can damage and pull hair, causing split ends and tearing.

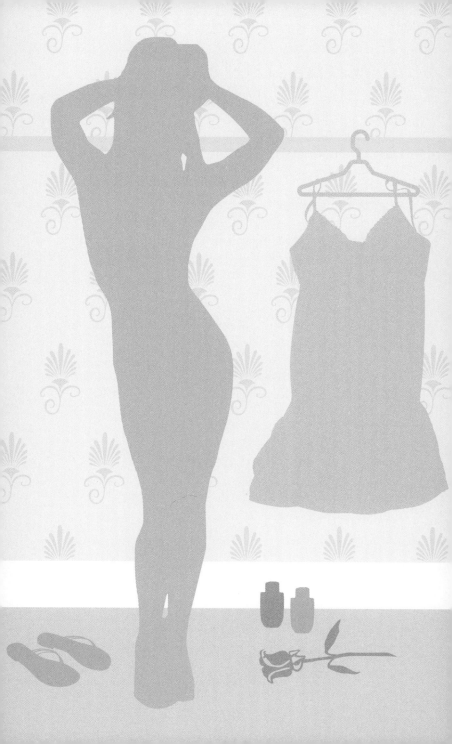

The Body Beautiful

CARING FOR YOUR BODY goes a long way to making you feel and look more beautiful, and just a little effort can achieve amazing results. On the following pages you will find body treatments and masks, home-spa ideas and salon secrets, cellulite busters and depilatory tips, as well as advice on everything from mani-pedis and massage to fragrances and fake tanning.

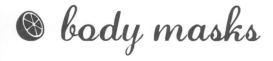# body masks

REVITALIZE WITH ROSE

Make a revitalizing body mask with rose and lime by mixing rosewater and lime juice with a little glycerine and use the lotion on dry skin after a bath. Store in the fridge if you want to keep it for more than a few days.

LOSE INCHES WITH CLAY

Clay products are great home spa choices for inch loss because they leach excess fluids out of the skin and help tone and tighten skin, especially if used with compressing bandages to squish cells together. The more absorbent the clay, the more inches will be lost.

GO NON-GREASY

Create a moisture-boosting, skin-conditioning body mask using witch hazel and olive oil, which will leave skin feeling great without making oily areas oilier. Apply just enough to soak in well.

PLAY DEAD

Dead sea salts are fantastic for replenishing skin health and boosting circulation. For the best results, add a handful to a warm bath, lie back and gently massage the skin to absorb the salty goodness.

MAKE YOUR OWN WRAP

The most simple wrap is clay with added salt, which is highly absorbent. Warm some water, add ingredients then dip in bandages and wrap yourself in them. You can add herbs such as rose petals, camomile or ginger powder, if required.

DON'T DRINK CAFFEINE

If you're having a body wrap, avoid caffeine, fried food, sugar and fizzy drinks for 24 hours before and after the treatment to boost its efficiency. All of these can add to toxin build-up and reduce the treatment's action.

BOOST CIRCULATION

If you're using a body mask, tighten up problem areas using gently wrapped plastic wrap or bandages, which can improve circulation by tightening the skin and helping it to release toxins.

GO FOR SEA CLAY

Sea clay is the best detoxifying product to help leach toxins out of the skin and boost circulation in underlying areas. For best results, use bandages or (old) towels to compress it onto the skin.

BATHE BEFOREHAND

If you're using a body mask or wrap at home, take a warm bath or shower beforehand to open pores and make the treatment more efficient at leaching toxins. Similarly, do the same before you visit the spa.

HOT AND COLD

Bath temperatures can be used therapeutically, but may not achieve the relaxing treat you are looking for. Cold baths reduce swelling by constricting blood vessels while hot ones relieve muscle soreness and eliminate body toxins.

GO FOR ALL-OVER RELAXATION

Don't forget to make sure you allow yourself time to wind down after a body treatment, as you may feel sleepy, or even dizzy or faint. Listen to your favourite music, read a book or have a cup of herbal tea. Allowing yourself to de-stress will prolong the effects of the experience.

FLUSH IT OUT

Drink lots of water before, during and after body masks to help remove toxins and stimulate the lymph system. This is especially important for detoxifying treatments, which are very dehydrating.

DRINK BE WARM

Choose a warm room for body masks and treatments so the mixture stays warm for longer and doesn't dry out. Warmer surroundings boost your circulation, which brings more blood to the surface and helps the mask do its work.

REST UP

Avoid exercise or anything that makes you sweat for 24 hours after you've had a body treatment or wrap because the sweat could interfere with the ongoing detoxification process. Take gentle exercise if you like but be careful not to overexert.

MAXIMIZE THE MASK

To maximize the effects of a detoxifying body mask, take a cool or lukewarm bath afterwards and then, two or three days later, take a hot bath which will open up the pores and release any accumulated toxins from the skin.

WRAP IN THE TUB

To avoid staining your bathroom with clay and other products, stand in the bath to apply your body mask or wrap. You can then easily wash away the excess product without mess.

body treatments

HOME SPA

To help keep it healthy and minimize the risk of illness, re-energize your body with a hydrotherapy bath. A warm bath can help revive joint and muscle pain, while a cold bath thins the blood, increases blood sugar and leaves the skin fresh and tingly.

ALWAYS REPLACE MOISTURE

Baths and showers always rob skin of its moisture, even if you use a very gentle body wash. Always use body oil or a specially formulated body lotion after bathing to replace lost moisture and keep skin hydrated.

HONEY HYDRATING WRAP

To rehydrate tired skin and replenish moisture, try a luxurious heated milk-and-honey body wrap at your favourite spa or salon. Honey acts as a natural humectant and the warm treatment will leave aching muscles thoroughly relaxed.

LIGHTEN UP

Darker areas of skin, as at the knees and elbows, are the result of very dry skin and accumulated skin cells. These will benefit from an intensive exfoliation treatment, followed by a rich moisturizing cream. To lighten skin at the elbows, cut a lemon in half and rub each half into an elbow.

WAX YOUR KNEES AND ELBOWS

The skin at the knees and elbows is prone to sagging and dryness as there are few oil glands there. Ease rough, cracked skin with a paraffin treatment. Used medically to aid aching joints, warm nutrient-rich paraffin is brushed on the area and allowed to harden before being removed. The treatment aids circulation, softens rough skin, cleanses the pores and loosens the joints.

THE WONDERS OF MESOTHERAPY

Mesotherapy involves the injection of vitamins, minerals and antioxidants into the middle layer of the skin. This is said to improve the quality and texture of the skin by replenishing essential vitamins that occur naturally within the cells.

FIRM UP FLABBY ARMS

Recognized as a fabulous treatment for cellulite, Velasmooth can work wonders on flabby arms. It involves three stages: infrared waves to boost metabolic rate; radio frequency waves that shock and tighten the skin, causing it to lift and contract; and suction to pummel the skin and draw out toxins. Several treatments may be needed for long-lasting results.

REJUVENATING BODY WRAP

Wrapping the body from chest to toes in a mineral rich mud or seaweed soaked cloth will invigorate tired skin, enhance circulation and help to detoxify, which will leave skin revitalized and glowing.

UPPER ARM FIRMER

The area directly above the outer elbow is one of the first places to show ageing saggy skin, yet it is often neglected because we never naturally see this part of our own body. It is also more resistant to the firming benefits of exercise than other parts as there are no large muscle groups there. To help, try massaging a firming body or face cream into the area.

FAT-BUSTING PLANTS

To stimulate the lymph flow and break down fatty tissue, natural plant extracts containing a combination of enzymes and nutrients can be injected into the middle layer of skin (mesoderm), using extremely small needles. A long-term course is recommended.

cellulite-busters

STRIDE AWAY CELLULITE

Walking is the best way to reduce cellulite, toning the muscles of the legs, hips and bottom and keeping heart rate gently elevated for fat reduction. Aim for at least 20 minutes brisk walking three or four times a week for best results.

PEEL OFF ORANGE PEEL

Eating oranges is a great way to reduce cellulite because of their high water content, which helps to plump skin. Other fruits containing high levels of water are also useful – try apples, grapefruit and tropical fruits like mango and pineapple.

UNDERSTAND ENDERMOLOGIE

Endermologie is a salon-based deep-tissue suction treatment that rolls and pinches fatty tissues to break down subcutaneous fat deposits, toxins and retained water. After a number of sessions, you should notice improvements in the overall texture and appearance of the skin.

DRY BRUSH DIMPLED SKIN

A favourite three-pronged method for dealing with cellulite is to first eliminate toxins from your diet, such as alcohol, caffeine and processed food, then to break it down by using dry skin brushing and lymphatic drainage massage and, finally, to firm up the skin with a good anti-cellulite tightening serum or body cream.

GET CAFFEINE TIGHTS

Invest in a pair of tights with added caffeine. The idea is that the temperature causes the release of caffeine microcapsules into the skin, increasing metabolic rate and the burning of fat to reduce cellulite.

MASSAGE IN DEEPLY

Always massage in a cellulite cream, working from the extremities towards the heart and in circular motions – it's the massaging effect that's as beneficial as the cream.

DETOX TO DUMP CELLULITE

Regardless of age, weight or body type all women can suffer from cellulite. Getting rid of unwanted toxins and waste will allow your liver to metabolize fats more efficiently and reduce cellulite. Undertake a seven-day detox plan, combined with body brushing and massage, and you should see visible results.

RESHAPE WITH HYPOXITHERAPY

Eliminate fat and cellulite from bottom and legs with a fat-burning treatment called Hypoxitherapy. Involving exercising and cycling under low atmospheric pressure, this increases blood supply and circulation and breaks down fatty deposits.

HIGH COLONIC CLEANSING

Constipation is one of the causes for toxins building up in your body and those toxins get trapped in connective tissue and appear as cellulite. Colonic cleansing, often used in conjunction with a detox, clears out the large intestine, killing harmful bacteria and parasites that live in the gut. It is a painless procedure performed by a therapist that also helps the colon absorb vitamins, minerals and essential fatty acids more efficiently.

SKIN-FOLD MASSAGE

Endermologie was developed in France to reduce the appearance of cellulite. Focusing on areas that are prone to the problem, such as saddlebag thighs, bottoms and tummies, a suction-roller device smoothes the skin surface and stimulates the circulation by eliminating toxins in the tissues.

CUT OUT CAFFEINE

Ingesting caffeine impairs circulation and lymph flow. Replace all caffeine drinks with detoxing green tea, dandelion tea or hot water with lemon and ginger.

DAILY BODY BRUSHING

Get into the habit of body brushing every day to slough off dead skin cells, boost circulation and encourage new regeneration. Skin will look smoother because better circulation helps disperse fatty deposits.

KNEAD AWAY LUMPS AND BUMPS

Vigorous massage will stimulate the circulation of the lymphatic drainage system and speed up toxin elimination. Target specific areas and simply massage in circular movements for a couple of minutes a day to help reduce cellulite. Alternatively, have a professional lymphatic drainage massage.

CIRCULAR BRUSHING STROKES

Using moderate pressure and short strokes with a natural bristle body brush, start brushing the skin in upwards circular movements from the lower body up towards the heart. As well as stimulating blood circulation in the tiny capillaries near the skin, it will tone and tighten the skin and help reduce cellulite deposits.

SCRUB UP

A very hot bath, around 32°C (90°F), will open the pores and encourage the body to sweat, helping to release harmful toxins.

IMPROVE LEGS WITH BIRCH OIL

Combat ugly cellulite with regular massage. Diet and exercise are all known to help reduce the lumpy orange-peel skin that appears at the top of the thigh and on the bottom, but massage using a plant-based cream like birch oil helps too by improving blood and lymph circulation, and releasing trapped toxins.

HAND MASSAGE FOR CELLULITE

Apply moisturizing cream to the area to be massaged and, using your thumb and forefingers, grip the skin and fatty layer beneath it and start to knead in small circular movements. Let your fingers glide smoothly over the skin and do not rub so hard that you bruise yourself.

TURN OFF THE HEAT

In the morning jump-start your body by gradually turning your warm shower water to cold. Let it run for a minute all over your face and body to give the lymphatic system a boost, and tone up the skin to leave it tingling.

NATURAL SALT SCRUBS

For an invigorating body scrub grab a handful of luxury salt granules, such as "Fleur de Sel", and mix them with a tablespoon of good-quality almond oil. Massage gently over rough skin, paying particular attention to knees and elbows, then rinse off with warm water.

WRAP UP WARM

After a warm detox bath, wrap up warmly in thick layers of clothes and your body will continue to sweat out toxins for another 30 minutes.

THREE MINUTES WITH A LOOFAH

Dry-brush your skin with a natural loofah first thing in the morning. You will feel the benefits as the accelerated blood flow invigorates you and sets your skin tingling – a great start to the day.

HEALTHY LIFESTYLE

Although firming creams can help lumpy orange-peel skin to look firmer, they cannot penetrate deep into the dermal layers to change the skin's structure so for best results ensure that you eat healthily and take adequate exercise.

SWEAT OUT TOXINS

Make your bathtime work for you by adding 450 kg (1 lb) of Epsom bath salts to the water. Epsom salts are made from the mineral magnesium sulfate, which draws toxins from the body, sedates the nervous system and relaxes tired muscles.

LASER LIGHT FIGHTS CELLULITE

Thought to temporarily reduce the appearance of cellulite, the Tri-Active laser combines suction massage to increase lymphatic drainage which filters fluid from the cells. Low-intensity diodes heat to stimulate collagen production and tighten the skin, which is left visibly smoother.

RIPPLES RESPOND TO TONING LIGHT

A successful Beverly Hills dermatologist has had good results on rippled cellulite using a device called the "Galaxie" which is usually used for wrinkles. Radio frequency and laser light energy are directed beneath the skin's surface, to stimulate the production of new collagen and tighten the skin.

REDUCE WATER RETENTION

Water retention contributes to the appearance of cellulite, but don't choose commercial diuretics as they can leach potassium from the body, contributing to osteoporosis. Natural diuretics are dandelion, nettle, astragalus, juniper, parsley and vitamin B6, but the best method is to radically reduce your intake of salt and increase your intake of water.

JUNK THE JUNK FOOD

Processed food contains artificial substances that the body finds hard to eliminate, and is a factor in the development of cellulite. Steer clear too of high-GI foods like white bread, rice and potatoes that raise levels of fat-storing insulin. Stick to a diet that contains natural and organic meats and vegetables, which are simply cooked.

SWEAT IT OUT

Cleanse the body by spending half an hour in a steam room. The heat increases metabolism and pulse rate, and as blood vessels become more flexible, the whole body benefits from better circulation, leaving you feeling relaxed and energized – and all without moving a muscle.

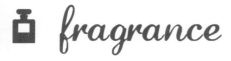 fragrance

STRIKE OIL
You can get perfume oils from health-food stores that smell exactly like some branded perfumes but cost a lot less. They tend to last much longer as well, due to the absence of alcohol.

SEARCH THE STORES
Different stores sell exactly the same branded bottle of perfume at different prices. And some may have special offers on your favourite, so always shop around to make savings and check the Internet.

JANUARY SALES
Stores bulk-buy perfumes before Christmas and so often have a surplus to get rid of in January. This is the best time to look for two-for-one and half-price offers. Other great dates are just after Valentine's Day or Mother's Day.

BE YOUR OWN PERFUMIER
Stir four to eight drops of your favourite essential oil into a little vodka. Leave for two days, then stir in 2 tablespoons of distilled water. Let it sit another couple of days before using it. The perfume can be stored in a dark-coloured glass bottle for six months.

PROLONG YOUR PERFUME
To help your favourite perfume retain its scent for longer, keep it away from damaging sunlight. Place it in its original box and store in a cool, dark place, such as a drawer.

BOUQUET OF ROSES
Make your own sweetly scented rose oil fragrance. Place three handfuls of dried rose petals into a glass jar with a screw-top lid. Pour in almond oil to within about 12 mm (½ in) of the brim. Put the jar in a pan of simmering water and leave in the water until the oil has removed all of the colour from the petals. Strain and decant in a lidded, dark glass container. Store for six months in a cool, dark place.

SCENTS AND SENSIBILITY

Don't wait until your favourite scent is all gone. When you start running low, find out if any friends or family are planning a trip abroad and ask them to get you some duty free. You'll often find that male friends have no plans to use their perfume allowance.

SIGNATURE SCENT

Studies show that men have more powerful memories of women who have a signature smell, so kick your addiction to bottle buying and stick to the one perfume that suits you, day and night. You will become more memorable (and better off!) instantly.

SCENT OF THE ORIENT

Some perfumes are very "heavy", while others are "light" and perfect for a sunny day. But if you choose a scent carefully, you can find one bottle that will be suitable for any time of day and whatever the weather. Oriental, also known as amber, scents tend to last longer and have the complex spicy notes needed to remain interesting.

THROW A PERFUME PARTY

We all have perfectly good perfumes that we're bored with. Instead of buying a new bottle, arrange for a few friends to gather up their unloved fragrances and host a perfume party.

WEAR IT NAKED

Don't just add perfume on your way out the door – it needs the warmth of your skin to activate the oils. Scent should be worn directly on your skin, under your clothes, for lasting effect. Put it on pulse points low on the body as it will rise with your body heat. Be like Marilyn Monroe and make Chanel No. 5 the only thing you wear to bed!

HAVE A NOSE ON THE NET

The Internet is usually the cheapest place to buy perfume as web-based companies don't have to cover the cost of store overheads in their prices. Just make sure it's a reputable site and that you're not buying a fake.

SINGLE LAYERS ONLY

Perfume brands encourage you to buy their full range of scented products including soap, shower gel and deodorant, by claiming that these extra items help layer the scent. However, provided you choose long-lasting perfume, it's fine to use cheap, unscented basics elsewhere on your body.

HEAVEN-SCENT SOAK

Down to your last few drops of perfume? Mix it with some baby oil and add to your bath for a soak that will leave your skin soft and beautifully scented.

DON'T DO DEPARTMENT STORES

Big stores are the prime destinations for perfume buyers, so they keep prices high. Try the supermarkets instead, as they tend to be far more competitive with pricing.

MISTRUST MISTS

Body sprays and mists don't last long. Their fragrance fades quickly so you'll have to keep refreshing it all day. Choose more concentrated perfumes that last longer and you won't have to apply them so often.

WAFT IN THE SCENT

Overdoing scent can be annoying to others, especially those next to you on public transport or at work. To ensure a beautiful, delicate application that's not overpowering, spray the fragrance into the air and walk through it – it will linger on your clothes and hair.

KEEP IT BOXED UP

Keeping perfumes in their boxes shields them from light, which can cause chemical changes in their make-up and helps them last longer than if exposed to light.

THROUGH THE WOODS

Chypre scents are based on mossy and fern notes that are often combined with jasmine, rose or citrus, and are ideal if you like warm, aromatic scents.

VIAL IT IN YOUR BAG

Invest in a small vial and decant some from the bottle if you want to carry scent around with you in your handbag, or choose a small travel size. If you take the whole bottle with you, and expose it to light or heat, the scent may go off prematurely.

BOTTLE COLLECTING

When you've used all of your special perfume, don't throw the bottle away. If it's a special-edition bottle (such as one produced for Christmas) it could become a collectors' item. Even within the first year some bottles have been known to increase by ten times in value.

DON'T BE A FOLLOWER

Love your friend's perfume? Don't rush out and buy it. Perfume reacts differently with an individual's skin, so it may not smell the same on you. Be sure to try her scent on your skin before making any rash and costly decisions.

BE CONSCIOUS OF COLOUR

Throw your perfume away if it changes colour (especially if it goes darker) or starts to smell different, as this means irreversible changes have taken place in the bottle, which could cause skin reactions.

GET SCENTS-IBLE

Perfume and scent can change the way you feel. To give yourself a lift, opt for citrus scents or vanilla, and for sexy evenings, try musk or rose.

DAYTIME FOR FLOWERS AND FRUIT

Traditionally the two fragrance families of florals and citrus are reserved for day. Florals are feminine and easy to wear, ranging from single notes to bouquets that include rose, lily of the valley, freesia and violet. Citrus is crisp, refreshing and tangy.

TEST ONLY FOUR

Don't try more than four scents at once, however tempting it is when trapped in a department store. You won't be able to differentiate between them, though sniffing coffee will help readjust your "nose".

A WATERFALL OF SCENT

The ozonic family of fragrances has watery notes that are often used to enhance floral, oriental and woody fragrances. If you like the fresh air feel of the seaside, these scents are right for you.

GET IN A DIFFERENT MOOD

Because most eau de toilettes are potent for only four to five hours, you can change fragrances throughout the day to suit your mood. Not many people have a "signature" scent they stick to for all occasions.

DON'T SPRAY ONTO SILK

While it is great to have your fragrance on your clothes and hair, avoid spraying directly onto fabric. Many materials, especially silk, will stain permanently.

COOL IS THE RULE

Prolong the shelf-life of your favourite fragrance by keeping it in the fridge. This will help preserve the ingredients, which can often be in delicate balance, and prevent scent changes.

TRY THIS LOTION NOTION

If your favourite scent doesn't have a matching body lotion, make your own by buying an unperfumed body lotion and adding a few drops of perfume. Make-up in small amounts to avoid it going off.

CHECK YOUR REACTIONS

Perfume is a common cause of allergies and skin reactions, which don't always happen in the exact area of application. If you think this might be the case, try cutting it out for a few days and see if the problem disappears. Avoid wearing any fragrance in the sun as it can cause rashes.

LIGHT OR HEAVY?

Choose your type of scent according to how you will wear it – eau fraîche only lasts for an hour or two; with eau de toilettes 20% of the scent will last all day; with eau de parfum 30% lasts all day; and with perfume 50% lasts all day.

A FLOWER GARDEN OF SCENTS

Learn to recognize the main flower scent behind the perfume – lily of the valley, one of the most delicate and sweetest flowers, is behind Christian Dior's Diorissimo and Jean Patou's Joy is based on a combination of jasmine and rose.

ORIENTAL FRAGRANCES

Spicy musks, woods and ambers form the basis of this sultry and seductive family of fragrances. They are heavier and longer lasting, making them popular for evening.

CARE IN THE WORKPLACE

If you love wearing perfumes, be thoughtful of others in the workplace or public spaces. Although you may love the scent, it can be a hazard for others, triggering asthma, migraine and other allergic reactions.

TAKE A BREAK

There is some evidence that sensitive skins can "get used" to a fragrance if worn every day, which could lead to skin reactions if you stop using it for a while and then start again. To prevent this problem, don't wear the same scent every day.

PHONE A FRIEND

If you wear the same scent most of the time, the chances are that your nose has adapted to the smell, which could lead to you using too much. If you've used the same scent for a year or more, ask a close friend to tell you honestly how strong your scent is on a scale of one (negligible) to ten (overpowering).

A NOSE FOR NEW SCENTS

When trying out a new scent, wait up to five hours for it to develop on your skin – this way you will first smell the top notes, then the middle at about two to four hours later (the important notes) and finally the full base note.

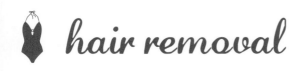

hair removal

TRY TURMERIC
The best natural depilatory is a turmeric paste, which gets rid of even thick hairs. Apply it before a bath, and leave it on to dry, then simply wash off for a naturally smooth look.

WARM UP INGROWING HAIRS
For ingrown pubic hairs along the bikini line, hold a hot compress against ingrown spots for ten minutes a couple of times a day to soften the skin and help the hairs work their way out.

POINT TO THE PROBLEM
Ingrown hairs on your bikini line, underarms or legs can be gently removed with a pair of pointed tweezers.

MAN, I FEEL LIKE A WOMAN
Women's razors tend to be more expensive than men's, so why not buy a men's razor? Although women's razors are probably prettier, men's ones tend to have more blades, which results in a closer shave.

BANISH BURN
You don't need store-bought post-shave balm to soothe razor burn. Simply rub honey onto your legs; aloe vera gel with a little witch hazel also works well.

MAKE YOUR OWN WAX
Stir the juice of a lemon and 50 ml (1.76 fl oz) of water in a pan. Add 225 g (8 oz) of sugar. Heat the mixture until it thickens. When the wax turns a darker colour take it off the heat and leave to stand. Be very careful to use only when it's cool enough to be applied.

DON'T OVERSOAK
Try not to soak in the bath too long before shaving or run the water too hot, as this causes skin to wrinkle and swell slightly, making a close, clean shave more difficult.

BIKINI MADE EASY

Nervous about waxing your own bikini line? The best wax to use is hard wax – it's made for coarse hair and "shrink-wraps" the hairs making them easier to pull out. After waxing press your hand down on your skin to relieve pain, and use tweezers to remove any hairs missed by the wax.

THE OUCH-FACTOR

If you are waxing your own upper lip, you can make the experience less painful by dabbing some oral gel (the kind used to relieve the pain of mouth ulcers and denture sores) from your medicine cabinet on the area first. It numbs the skin and makes the whole process far less painful.

BRAVING THE COLD

Doing a perfect do-it-yourself job using cold wax is easier than you think. Simply smooth the strips onto your leg in the direction of hair growth. Hold the skin above the strip taut. Pull the strip off quickly in the opposite direction of the hair growth. It's less messy than hot waxing but just as cheap!

BE A SWEETIE

To make your own sugaring paste, mix eight parts sugar with one part water and one part lemon juice. Heat until smooth and thick. Leave to cool until it can be spread easily and thinly.

HOT WAX LIKE A PRO

Apply heated wax in the direction of hair growth. Wax section by section, rather than covering the entire leg. Press the cloth strip firmly over the wax, hold your skin taut and pull off quickly against the hair growth.

TO POINT OR ANGLE?

If you're plucking areas like the eyebrow, chin or upper lip, choose angled tweezers for targeted hair removal – the slant makes it easier to grasp and pluck in the direction of hair growth, which reduces soreness and redness. Pointed tweezers should be used to extract very short hairs.

WAXING LYRICAL

Don't be embarrassed by upper lip hair – be embarrassed about spending a fortune on salon waxes. For a tenth of the price you can be fuzz-free for months using a shop-bought facial wax strip kit.

PAIN-FREE HAIR REMOVAL

Why pay for painful hair removal when you can bleach unwanted body and facial hair at home? It's easy, pain-free and affordable, plus you won't get unsightly ingrown hairs.

A SUGAR SOLUTION

Sugaring is often a better choice than waxing if you have somewhere to go afterwards, as wax can stick to legs but the sugar solution is water soluble, which means it wipes off, leaving no telltale marks. Sugar waxing works in exactly the same way as traditional waxing but because the solution is sugar-based, it dissolves in water, so there is no sticky residue to clean from your skin.

EXFOLIATE BEFORE YOU WAX

To avoid ingrown hairs post-waxing, remove dead skin cells, which might obstruct the hair beforehand by exfoliating the area to be waxed. Because skin will be softer, you are less likely to develop ingrown hairs.

GO FLAT FOR LARGE

For large areas of hair removal, such as touching up patches on legs or arms which have been missed with waxing, use flat-headed tweezers, which can pull more than one hair out at a time and make plucking more efficient and quicker. Remember to always pluck in the direction of hair growth, so make sure the hairs are all growing in the same direction.

CALM DOWN WITH CAMOMILE

Many spas use camomile wax, which is normal wax infused with calming camomile, which can ease pain and redness following waxing. If you have sensitive skin, this can mean happier hair removal – ask your beautician for advice.

BLEACH AWAY DOWN

If you have downy hair on your forehead or in front of your ears, rub a freshly cut lemon over the hair and leave for five to ten minutes before rinsing off for a natural bleaching agent which won't make them bright white.

WAIT AND SEE

If you have ingrown pubic hairs, don't be tempted to over exfoliate as this could cause further skin trauma, which may result in sore spots, infections or more serious irritation of the skin. Wait until it's gone and then exfoliate.

SHAKE AND WAX

When waxing your hair at home, first shake talcum powder over the area to be waxed as this helps the strip to rip and be more effective.

DON'T RUB RED SPOTS

If you have red spots caused by ingrown hairs or sore patches following hair removal on your bikini line, wear loose-fitting underwear and clothing until the bumps are gone to avoid friction.

POP A PILL

If you find the pain of waxing or epilating too much to bear, lessen the pain by taking paracetamol or ibuprofen 15 minutes beforehand to help reduce your suffering.

GET IT ALL OUT

When waxing, sugaring or plucking, be sure to pull the hair out by the roots by pulling in the direction of hair growth in smooth, even pulls. Do not allow the hair to break below the skin surface, which can lead to rough regrowth and ingrown hairs.

BEWARE OF WAXING

If you are using Retin-A, Accutane or other skin-exfoliating medications, you should tell your beautician before your waxing appointment as this can cause increased skin sensitivity. The therapist may decide to modify the treatment accordingly.

DON'T WAX ON SUNBURN

Laser peels and sunburn are two big no-nos for waxing. Because both procedures expose the more sensitive layers of the skin and can cause redness and heat retention in skin layers, you should avoid waxing within a week of either of them.

CONDITION AND SHAVE

If you have run out of shaving foam, use hair conditioner when shaving legs. Because it's smooth, it will stop the skin dragging and help you shave smoothly without stretching the skin.

KEEP IT TO YOURSELF

Never be tempted to use someone else's razor or let them use yours. It could open you up to the chances of infection because it's so close to the skin's surface and there's the risk of cutting and nicking skin.

REDUCE FACIAL HAIR WITH ROSE

Stimulating facial hair will cause it to grow more. To keep it unstimulated, use a light toner like rosewater and a light moisturizer that won't nourish the hair root.

BE A WATER BABY

To ensure an extremely close shave, soften hairs first by having a short, warm bath as this is a great way to hydrate before shaving and hair is easier to cut when wet and supple.

KEEP YOUR COOL

Avoid saunas, hot baths, exercise or sunbathing for 24 hours after waxing. All of these can raise your body temperature, which means you may sweat more, causing irritation to treated areas.

LASER HAIRS AWAY

For permanent hair loss, laser removal is most effective where there is high contrast between the hair and skin colour, such as dark-haired people with pale skin.

WET SHAVE FOR SMOOTH SKIN

As any barber will tell you, wet shaves are the most effective. Before shaving, wet the hair as well as the skin, use a foam or mousse specifically for shaving, and pull the skin taut to ensure a smooth finish. Work upwards with long, even strokes.

TAKE IT ON THE SHIN

The skin on the shin is especially thin and prone to becoming dry, wrinkled and flaky if neglected, so pay special attention when shaving this area and slather on a moisturizer every morning, through the whole year, to keep legs smooth.

SMOOTH AND BARE

If you want to remove body hair on a long-term basis, try IPL (intense pulsed light) treatments. IPL devices rely on the absorption of light energy, which is targeted at the hair follicle, disabling it and preventing further growth. You will need several treatments, as hair has to be treated during its growing stage.

LASER BEAM REMOVAL

This treatment is best suited to light-skinned people with dark hair because the melanin pigment in the hair absorbs the laser light making it more effective. The procedure causes the temperature within the hair shaft and follicle to rise, effectively killing it.

GET TRIM

Trimming hair with nail scissors before waxing makes the job a lot easier, avoids tangles and can reduce pain. You'll also be able to make sure you get straight lines to avoid that uneven look.

SHADY LADY

Laser treatment is the best solution for removing dark hair growth on the upper lip. Choose a long-pulse laser (Alexandrite) in preference to the more common IPL (intense pulse light) for the most effective results.

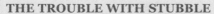

THE TROUBLE WITH STUBBLE

Hormonal changes in the body usually mean an increase in unwanted facial hair on the upper lip and sides of the face that has to be dealt with. Tweezers are brilliant for eyebrow plucking, but are much too severe to rip out tiny facial hairs so are best avoided for these.

WAX AWAY

Shadowy upper lips need to be treated regularly, and if you have dark colouring it's best to get a hot wax treatment at a salon. This will remove the small hairs instantly, but it can be painful and will leave your skin temporarily irritated.

DISSOLVING PROBLEMS

For facial hair, you will need to use a depilatory cream or gel specially formulated for this delicate area. Quick to work and inexpensive, these react with the protein structure of the hair, so that the hair dissolves and is removed from the skin's surface. However, they can irritate sensitive skin so do a patch test first.

LOW-LEVEL ELECTROLYSIS

This treatment takes lots of time, and is painful but permanent. It must be performed by a qualified electrologist, who inserts a needle into the follicle and then sends an electric current to kill it. If performed badly inflammation and scarring may occur.

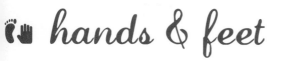# hands & feet

TAKE OUT TOBACCO STAINS

Rub tobacco-stained fingers and nails with half a freshly cut lemon for five to ten minutes to help bleach skin naturally without drying it out. Rubbing the back of the hands with lemon will also fade age spots.

SUN-PROTECT YOUR HANDS

In summer, add a layer of sunscreen to your hands or use a hand cream with SPF to protect skin against dryness, wrinkles and premature ageing.

ZESTY HEEL SCRUB

There's no need to buy expensive foot creams to shift rough skin on your heels. Instead, simply cut a lemon in half, squeeze out the juice and fill with sugar. Place the lemon over your heel and rub firmly.

SOLE SEARCHER

Another cost-effective way to remove hard, dead skin from your feet is to add rock salt to a little olive oil and use as a scrub. Afterwards, moisturize with warm olive oil.

TEA-RRIFIC TOOTSIES

If your feet are prone to smelling less than fragrant sometimes, there's no need to buy specialist products. The tannins in tea fight odour-causing bacteria, so to avoid stinky soles, soak your feet in cooled, strong black or green tea for several minutes before patting dry.

FEELING FRUITY?

To exfoliate your hands and to help reduce age spots, mix the juice of two fresh limes and 225 g (8 oz) of sugar together. Rub into your hands, leave for three to five minutes, then rinse with warm water and pat dry.

FUNGUS-FREE FEET

Medicine for toenail fungus isn't cheap and doesn't always work. So treat your feet by soaking them in a mixture of equal amounts of white vinegar and water for 30 minutes daily until the condition clears.

BEST FOOT FORWARD

There's no need to go to the beauty salon to have a softening pedicure treatment; do it yourself. Pour 750 ml (25.4 fl oz) of full-fat milk into a bowl and soak your feet. It will leave your skin supersoft.

SMOOTHING SOCKS

Expensive moisturizers aren't the only way to fight dry, chapped skin. Mash a banana with a little honey, lemon juice and margarine to make a moisturizing paste. Smear on your feet and wear cotton socks to bed. Wash off in the morning and feel how unbelievably smooth your soles are.

GET SOME WRIST ACTION

To ease tired hands and give yourself a circulation boost, hold both hands in front of you with palms facing inwards, loosen their wrist grip and flap them backwards and forwards. Feel them tingle as the blood rushes to them.

KNOW THE BACK OF YOUR HAND

The skin on the back of your hand is an excellent way to test for dehydration. Pinch it and count how long it takes to return to being smooth. If it's more than a second, your skin's telling you that you need to drink more water.

SCRUB WELL

Mix a paste of almond oil and salt in the palm of one hand and use
to scrub the back of your hands and over your knuckles – your hands
will feel and look silky smooth.

GO HAND IN GLOVE

Prevent problems by wearing rubber gloves when washing dishes and
doing other household chores. Keep exposure to harsh chemicals,
especially bleach, to a minimum.

BOWL HANDS OVER

For hands that are smooth and wrinkle free, soak them in a bowl of
warm water for five minutes before drying and applying your favourite
hand cream. The water soaks into the skin and the cream forms a
barrier, locking it in and easing aches and pains at the same time.

SLEEP ON THE JOB

For an overnight treat for hands that will moisturize and firm skin,
slather on a generous layer of rich hand cream, then put on a pair of
gloves and leave overnight.

GIVE A TIGHT SQUEEZE

If you have dry finger ends, hang nails or flaky, ridged nails, give
them a boost by squeezing the tip of each finger as hard as possible
for about five seconds to activate blood circulation into the nail bed.

KEEP CREAM TO HAND

Do as all the beauty editors do and keep hand cream by all your taps
(faucets) so it's easy to reapply cream whenever you wash.

STAY OUT OF HOT WATER

The repeated use of soap and water damages the top layer of the skin
and can cause chapping. Avoid strong soap and hot air dryers, and opt
for lukewarm water rather than the hot tap alone.

KEEP HANDS YOUNG

Take care of your hands before they give away your secrets. Hand skin is frequently neglected, but it's often the real telltale sign of age. Invest in a rich hand cream day and night to keep your hands looking young and tender.

DON'T RAZOR IT OFF

Never remove hard skin with a razor blade, or allow nail technicians or pedicurists to use one on you. This will only spur the skin into producing harder skin to replace it, which defeats the purpose of having it removed. Your therapist may use a strong exfoliator scrub or solution to aid in the removal of tough skin.

PUMICE AWAY HARD SKIN

To remove hard skin on feet, rub with a pumice after soaking the feet for at least ten minutes to soften problem areas, such as the balls of the feet and the heels. The natural stone will not only remove dead skin but will boost circulation to the area, encouraging regeneration.

BE A BAREFOOT BEAUTY

Allow feet to breathe and you'll avoid many unsightly problems like fungal infections. Use natural, breathable fibres whenever possible for socks and try to go barefoot for at least an hour a day.

TREAT ATHLETE'S FOOT WITH TEA TREE

Tea tree oil, with its naturally astringent and antibacterial properties, can help prevent the spread of athlete's foot by drying out skin and making it hard for the fungus to spread.

ORANGE IS THE AGENT

Massage feet with orange oil, which will help draw out toxins and impurities from the skin and boost the regeneration of cells. Rub the ball of the foot in a circular motion, and work your way down the sides to the heel.

PEP UP WITH PEPPERMINT

Invigorate the tired skin of your feet and lower legs with products
infused with essential oils of peppermint and eucalyptus, which have
been shown to have revitalizing effects. Or choose an unscented
product and add your own.

COOL WITH MANGO

Cool hot, burning or swollen feet with mango juice, which rejuvenates
skin as well as reducing the pain and discomfort of problem feet. Soak
feet for a few minutes or apply with cotton wool before a warm bath.

GET FEET FIT

Keep feet and toes flexible by standing and walking on tiptoe whenever
you can. And practise picking up pencils or marbles with your toes.

SALT AWAY STIFFNESS

If you have stiff, sore or aching hands, soak them in salt water for
15–20 minutes, then rinse with fresh water. This will help reduce
swelling and restore the fluid balance.

BAN WARTS WITH DANDELION

Dandelion stems have long been believed to help banish warts. Apply
the juice of a dandelion stem two or three times daily for several weeks.

SOCK IT TO DRY FEET

Before bed, exfoliate feet and rub in cream or oil, then pull on a pair
of socks to help them make the most of their newfound moisture all
night long. When you wake up, they'll be as soft as a baby's!

NEVER SHARE SHOES

Other people's shoes, especially if they're well-worn favourites, will have
moulded to their feet, which could cause you problems if you borrow
them by putting pressure on areas which might not be used to it.

SEE YOUR PODIATRIST

If you're suffering corns or callouses, see a podiatrist, also called a chiropodist, who is skilled in dealing with all kinds of foot problems, from verrucas to deformities, and will do more than a pedicurist to help you solve these problems. They will also assess how you walk and the shape of your foot to see if there are any physical reasons for the cause of your problems, and be able to advise and provide surgery for persistent ingrown nails.

WEAR THE RIGHT SHOE SIZE

Squeezing your feet into too-small shoes can cause long-term problems as corns and callouses build-up on pressured areas, and areas of dry skin build up to help protect the feet against shoe pressure. Fit and buy shoes in the afternoon when your feet are the most swollen and remember that air travel and pregnancy will make feet swell.

HANDS HATE WATER

Because the skin is thin and endlessly ravaged by the elements, keep your hands dry as much as possible. Water left on hands will evaporate leaving them dried up and red. Use a hand cream that contains lanolin.

OLD LADY HANDS

A salon-inspired handcare treatment that includes a self-heating exfoliant to skim off dry flaky skin, followed up by a luxuriant hand cream to put back softness, will make a noticeable difference to wrinkled hands.

CHANGE IT AROUND

Don't wear the same shoes for more than a few days running – your feet will begin to adapt to wearing them and you may get problems in pressured areas. Switch between flats and heels, and round and pointed toes regularly.

BE A BAREFOOT BEAUTY

For general foot health, try to reduce the amount of time you spend in shoes. At your work desk or at home, use every opportunity to slip off your footwear and walk around barefoot. This is particularly important if you are trying to prevent such conditions as bunions or calluses.

CHOOSE MILD SOAP

If you wash your hands as often as you should, make sure you are using a good-quality soap with natural ingredients like lemon or oatmeal. Cheap soaps leave hands dry and chapped.

FOOT MASSAGE

A weekly home massage with a massage oil can not only help reduce any pain from years of accumulated stress on the feet, but it can soothe and hydrate rough skin and increase circulation to the extremeties.

FEELING LIVERISH

Over-the-counter skin lighteners work by inhibiting the natural pigment called melanin which lies deep in the skin with an active ingredient called hydroquinone. It may take weeks for the new lightened skin cells to reach the surface and liver spots to reduce, but it does work.

 # nails too long?

SHAPE SHIFTER

You don't need to visit a salon to make your nails look groomed. You can make square nails appear more elegant by applying polish down the centre only. Pale shades are best for short nails or stubby hands, while darker shades make chunky hands look delicate.

NAIL ART NAILED

With a little practice you can apply nail art to your own nails. Once you have covered your nails in a base colour and allowed to dry, draw patterns using an old lipstick brush and a different colour of polish.

GET SALON SAVVY

Next time you get your nails done at a salon ask for the "shape and polish" rather than a full manicure. They usually cost a quarter of the price and unless your cuticles are in really bad shape the end result will be identical.

MAXIMIZE NAIL GROWTH

To stimulate nail growth, massage the base of the nails with cuticle oil several times a day. This will stimulate and nourish the nail bed, encouraging new growth.

HEAT UP YOUR NAILS

Bend the fingers of the hands in towards the palms and rub the nails for a minute to give your nails a boost of oxygen and nutrient-rich blood, which will reduce nail problems.

AIM FOR A PERFECT 10

Don't assume your nine perfect nails will hide the chipped one. If it's small, fill in the chip with a quick coating of colour but if larger re-do the colour on the whole nail.

DO KEEP NAILS NEAT

You don't need to spend lots of money on a weekly manicure for pretty hands. Just make sure they're moisturized and your nails are a neat oval shape. Instead of always applying polish, invest in a nail buffer for natural gloss. It costs next to nothing and lasts for years.

COOL TREATMENT

Yogurt is as good as any pre-manicure conditioning treatment for hands and nails. Simply combine 225 g (8 oz) of natural (plain) yogurt with the juice of an apple. Refrigerate for several hours and then use to massage your hands and nails. Rinse the excess off afterwards.

CUTER CUTICLES

If you have dry, ragged cuticles, don't turn to expensive cuticle creams for help. Instead, rub leftover avocado skins into your cuticles and leave for 30 minutes. The vitamin E and natural oils in this fruit will help your fingers heal.

JUICY SKIN SOFTENER

To make a delicious-smelling cuticle softener, blend 1 teaspoon of papaya or mango juice with ½ teaspoon of egg yolk and 1 teaspoon of cider vinegar. Apply to cuticles and leave for as long as possible before rinsing.

BACK TO LIFE

If your nail polish has dried up there's no need to throw it out. Just add a tiny drop of nail polish remover, shake the bottle and it's as good as new.

EXTEND YOUR RANGE

If you have difficulty growing all your nails to the same length, fake it with extensions. Gel versions are glued onto the real nail, then cut and shaped. These are less irritating than acrylic versions, which are longer lasting and stronger but more difficult to remove.

GO SOFT, NOT LOOSE

The excessive use of nail hardeners that contain formaldehyde can cause lots of nail problems, including peeling, splitting and loose nails, when the nail plate separates from the nail bed. If you suspect this is the source of your problems, go easy on products and use a perfume-free nail cream.

HERO HERB

You can use garlic to make your nails stronger instead of expensive nail-strengthening treatments. Add 1 tablespoon of finely chopped fresh garlic to a bottle of clear nail polish. Leave the bottle for one week and then apply as needed. Don't worry – your nails won't smell and they will be far less likely to split and break.

HARD AS NAILS

For weak or brittle nails, apply a nail strengthener every day for a week, then remove and leave the nails to rest for a few days before repeating for another week, if necessary. Make sure you file the nails into a square shape rather than an oval, which will avoid weakening the sides and causing splits and tears.

HANG TEN

If the nails are frequently immersed in water, the outer skin layer may split away from the cuticle causing painful splits or hangnails. Snip off with clean scissors, or prevent problems from occurring by keeping the skin soft with regular applications of moisturizing hand cream.

PRIME NAILS WITH PROTEIN

When nails easily crack or break they can be a permanent worry. Weak nails may be caused by a protein deficiency in the diet. Increase nutritional intake by eating more lean meat, fish, fresh fruit and vegetables and use a nail cream to help hydrate.

BASE, COLOUR AND TOP

Always follow the three-step programme to varnish your nails: first apply a base coat to protect the nail from discolouring, then apply two coats of the colour, and finish with a clear, glossy top coat for extra shine and to guard against chips.

NICE GIRLS DON'T BITE

To help you stop biting your nails, visit a nail bar each week or every other week. When your nails are nicely filed and varnished, you're less likely to bite them. And if your hands look beautiful, you're less likely to want to cover them up (as most nail-biters tend to do).

MEND A BROKEN NAIL

Nail patches are tiny adhesive strips that bring the two sides of a split back together again. They are best applied by a professional manicurist, though there are over-the-counter versions.

SILK FOR STRENGTH

For nails that repeatedly break or are soft, visit a salon for a silk-wrapping treatment. A thin layer of silk is glued to the nails and buffed into an invisible finish.

CARRY IT OFF

Carry your nail polish with you so you can touch up nails if they chip en route. If this sounds too high maintenance, use a clear shade of gloss, which, if it chips, won't show.

FILE FIRST

For at-home manicures, file first before you remove old nail varnish. The polish keeps the nail protected and if you use a remover first, the nail will be weakened and softer.

DO THE DIP TIP

To speed up nail varnish drying, run nails under cold water for ten minutes to help the varnish form a hard, knock-free coating in no time at all.

BREAK FREE OF BRITTLE NAILS

Brittle nails can be caused by over-exposure to the sun, a poor diet or the prolonged use of commercial nail hardeners. Avoid the use of hardeners or varnishes containing formaldehyde, which has a drying effect on nails.

CARE FOR CUTICLES

Massage a cuticle oil or cream into the base of the nails at least once a day to prevent dryness, scarring and hangnails. If cuticles are damaged and painful, gently apply a moisturizer twice daily until they heal.

BUFF AWAY RIDGES

Ridges on the nail are mostly down to genetics but although you can't change them, you can smooth the ridged nail surface with a buffer and buffing cream.

CHECK YOUR IRON LEVELS

If you've recently developed ridges on your nails, which you haven't suffered before, it could be a sign of anaemia and you should consult your doctor. On the other hand, it might be the result of an over-zealous manicurist, so don't panic just yet!

SEAL IN DRY NAILS

To protect nails from drying, use a waterproof varnish that seals moisture in the nail and repels water and dirt. A waxy lip balm or nail oil can also be quite effective at moisturizing nails overnight.

LET YOUR NAILS BREATHE

Leave nails unpainted for at least a few days a month to help them breathe. This will reduce yellowing and staining from polish on the nail and give it a chance to recover health and glow.

BACK TO BASES

If you have yellow nails, it could be because you haven't used a base coat underneath your regular nail colour. Yellow patches or streaks that don't go away could be due to fungal infections that might need treatment.

FILE WITHOUT FRICTION

When filing nails, work in one direction from the outside edge toward the centre, rather than sawing back and forth, as too much friction can cause splits and tears. Angle the file slightly so you are filing away more from underneath the nail than on top. Avoid metal emery boards, which can be too harsh for nail ends.

TWINKLE THOSE TOES

Pale, subtle varnishes are wasted on summer toenails – open-toed sandals cry out for bright colours, such as shocking pink, or sparkly and metallic hues.

LET SPOTS GROW OUT

White spots on nails are usually the result of trauma to the nail or nail bed. Give the spots time to grow out and make an effort to be gentle when manicuring your nails – prodding beneath the cuticles, where new growth is generated, can cause white spots and damaged nails.

LIGHTEN UP WITH LEMON

Lighten discoloured nails with a whitening scrub containing a mild abrasive or with a remover containing lemon juice to bleach out colour. Ask your local manicurist or chemist for product recommendations.

CHILL OUT

Nail varnish will stay fresher for longer if it's kept in the refrigerator, which will help prevent it separating and clogging due to heat and light damage.

GORGEOUSLY GROOMED NAILS

The strongest type of artificial nails are acrylics and gels. The manicurist has to roughen up your own nail surface before painting over thin layers of liquid acrylic, which is extended up above your natural nail to the desired length. Easy to paint and strong enough to last for around three weeks, they make ugly hands look beautiful.

ELEGANCE AT YOUR FINGERTIPS

If your nails are on the short side, give an illusion of length by leaving a narrow strip of bare nail on each side when applying varnish. This will instantly narrow your nails.

WHITEN YOUR TIPS

If you haven't got time to paint your nails, fill in the underside of nail tips with a white nail pencil, which can give a naturally glamorous boost to unpainted nails.

CLING ON

Wait at least 45 minutes after painting your toenails before putting on closed-toe shoes, but if you absolutely must go out, wrap your toes in plastic wrap before slipping on shoes to avoid smudges.

BE A SQUARE

Clip and file toenails squarely in line with the ends of the toes so that the growth does not push into the surrounding tissue, which can be ugly and painful.

PAINT LIKE A PRO

To help nails look long and strong, start the polish in a curve in line with, and just above, the cuticle. Avoid getting polish on the cuticle, which shortens nails. If you slip, use a cotton bud to remove excess polish.

QUICK-FIX SPLITS

Never leave the house with a tiny split or tear in your nails, as it is bound to develop into a ripped or broken nail with time. Use an over-the-counter nail mender kit and apply a tiny strip of fibrous paper over the split before painting nail-mending liquid onto it and covering with polish.

ZAP FLECKS WITH ZINC

White flecks in the nails are caused by injury or, in some cases, a deficiency of zinc. Supplement your diet with eggs, shellfish, chickpeas and lentils, all good sources of dietary zinc.

OPT FOR ACETONE-FREE

To remove nail varnish, choose an acetone-free remover, which will lift off the colour without drying or damaging the nail surface. Acetone removers can strip nails of natural oils, making them dry and dull.

DON'T CUT CUTICLES

Instead of cutting cuticles, which can cause them to become hard and scarred, soak hands and push them back with a flannel or towel, then apply a cuticle oil or cream to keep them soft.

SMOOTH OUT NAILS

To avoid ridges and irregularities in the nail surface, apply a base coat before nail varnish or colour, which will also provide a protective layer and prevent staining.

THINK THIN

Polish that peels from the edge of the nail is usually due to the layers having been too thickly applied. Rather than one or two thick coats, try larger numbers of thinner coats instead.

COLOUR THAT LASTS

Colour wears off the tips of polished nails first. To make your manicure last longer, take the colour over the edge of the nail to underneath – the added polish will protect against chipping.

FAKE IT

Don't let ugly broken toenails ruin your summer look when they will be constantly exposed in strappy sandals. Fake plastic nails that are glued onto your own nails at home and then shaped to the right size are perfect for toes that are unlikely to be inspected at close range.

ALWAYS ON SHOW

Well-groomed nails will always get noticed. Clear or pale pink varnish will give you a chic, finished look that is much better than long red talons which are ageing and brash.

FEED NAILS FOR GROWTH

As you age your nails grow at about half the rate they did when you were younger. Feed them by massaging a vitamin-rich oil into the base of the nails every night to encourage growth from the nail bed.

A BUFF TOO FAR

Nude nails that are clean, shiny and buffed are preferable to a single coat of chipped polish, but only buff nails once a week. Over-buffing weakens the nails by taking away the top layer, and making them more porous.

LONGER- LOOKING NAILS

If you want to avoid smudged and bleeding varnish, leave a margin around the nail when applying. It will also make your nails look longer and thinner too.

KEEP NAILS HYDRATED

The health of nails and hair is very closely related to the overall health of the body. Keep the cuticle hydrated with specially formulated cuticle oil or a greasy lip balm, which can double up as instant moisture.

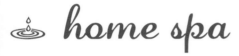 *home spa*

GET SPOTLESS WITH A SPONGE

For the best non-traumatic face cleansing experience, choose a small natural sea sponge and use small circular motions to work softly over the skin of the face and neck. This will ensure thorough washing without cleansing. Natural sea sponges are softer and last longer than synthetic versions and they don't absorb odour.

STEAM ROOM

Create your own steam room by closing the door and window in your bathroom and turning on the shower. Your skin will be warmed and primed for further treatment, such as pumicing, pedicures and manicures or body and hair masks.

WAX IN MOISTURE

Give yourself a home wax pedicure by melting paraffin wax in the microwave to create a wax bath. Moisturize feet well and dip into the wax three times, allowing each layer to dry. The wax should feel warm but not hot. Set for 20 minutes and peel off.

PAMPER WITH PATCHOULI

Add a few drops of essential oils to a cup of hot water while you bathe to infuse the room with healing properties. Choose patchouli for lifting the spirits or neroli and ylang-ylang for re-balancing.

COMPRESS STRESS

Make a quick stress-relieving compress by adding a few drops of lavender or camomile essential oil to a bowl of warm water and soaking a cotton cloth in it for five minutes, then apply to the face and neck as a compress and breathe deeply. Repeat three times.

REJUVENATE WITH JUNIPER

If you want a home spa experience to stimulate your circulation and invigorate tired muscles and minds, try adding essential oils of basil and juniper to your bathing experience. They have been shown to have stimulating effects and can pep you up for a good start to the day or right before an important meeting.

GET A GOMMAGE

For a home spa gommage (salt glow) as good as any salon, mix ground sea salt with 12 drops of a stimulating essential oil such as grapefruit, lemon or thyme. Make a paste by adding enough water to spread easily and apply in brisk circular strokes, especially on hips and thighs.

TRY CYROTHERAPY

Steal a salon secret (cyrotherapy is extreme cold applied for therapeutic purposes) for your own home – after applying a face-firming treatment, place an ice cube inside a small plastic bag and gently rub over the face and eye area for several minutes to plump up and tone the skin.

SCENT-SATIONAL PLEASURE

An essential oil diffuser will add to the overall effect of the at-home spa experience. Choose either a relaxing oil such as lavender or an invigorating one like rosemary, according to your mood. Play a CD of nature sounds, turn off all phones and retreat from the world for a few hours.

GLISTEN WITH GLYCERINE

For a home treatment for dry skin, mix glycerine with lemon juice and rosewater, in equal parts, and use it as a moisturizer or face mask to smooth out lines and plump up dehydrated areas.

COPY CLEOPATRA

Cleopatra was famous for her smooth skin and milk baths. Follow her beauty secret by adding 3 cups of powdered milk or fresh milk to a warm bath. The lactic acid in the milk will soften and gently exfoliate skin.

GARDEN HERB SOAK

Place a bunch of garden herbs such as rose, lavender and rosemary in a tea strainer and hang it from the running tap in your bath for a healing soak from your own botanical garden!

LIVE THE FANTASY

Lie back in the tub and float away with a fantasy that you are somewhere exotic. Visualizations like this have been shown to help relaxation by releasing feel-good chemicals in the bloodstream.

SOME LIKE IT NOT HOT

For a relaxing bath, make sure the water is pleasantly warm rather than hot, which can stimulate your system and cause the skin to slacken and dehydrate as a result. Always test the water before you enter.

HAVE A HOME VISIT

Many beauty therapists and stylists will visit your home to deliver a personal and private haircut, manicure or other beauty treatment, bringing all their own equipment, including a massage bed.

BUBBLE BATH

Many bubble baths and foams can be extremely drying, so if you are planning to have a long soak, make sure the formula includes softening oils in the ingredients list, or else add an oil, such as sweet almond oil, to a ready-prepared solution for extra-moisturizing results.

massage

TOOL UP
Use wooden or plastic self-massage tools, such as balls, rollers and bongers, while you're in the bath to promote relaxation. The added benefit of the warm water helps to make massage more effective, especially if you're trying to unknot tense muscles.

BE A TENNIS PRO
Instead of shelling out for an expensive salon massage, make your own back relaxer by lying on your back on a couple of used tennis balls, positioned at the top of your buttocks or your lower back, with your knees pointing up and your feet flat on the floor. Then roll around to release tension in the back area.

GET YOUR HAND IN
Give yourself a circulation mini-boost when applying hand cream by using small circular movements to rub the cream into your knuckles and joints. Use your thumbs to massage the backs of your hands.

KNEAD BETWEEN THE LINES
Reduce forehead lines caused by tension by using a soft, shallow pinch to relax muscles. Make your hand into a fist, then pinch skin between your thumb and index finger for gentle stimulation.

BREAST UPLIFT
The thin skin on your breasts is prone to sagging and toxin build-up. Massage problems away using almond oil and gentle sweeping strokes from the underside up into your armpits.

MAKE THE MOST OF OIL

Use oil during massage to avoid dragging skin and causing it to sag and stretch. Small amounts applied first to the hands are best, as that will ensure you don't use too much.

SIT UP FOR A GREAT FACE

For facial massages, sit upright or recline rather than stand or lie flat on your back. This will help you breathe evenly and deeply and keep muscles relaxed.

FINISH WITH A BATH

After your massage, soak in a bath for a ten-minute relaxation. Aromatherapy oils are particularly beneficial at this time because you will already be relaxed and have stimulated skin, which will make the oils more efficient.

NURTURE YOUR NECK

With your right hand, gently massage the left side of your neck at the shoulder in a rhythmic motion, working from the base to the ear, and moving slightly round to the back as you do so, in circular strokes. Repeat on the right side of the neck using your left hand. Finish with the fingers of both hands working either side of the spine at the back of your neck.

CONSIDER THE SINUS POINTS

Massaging the sinus points helps reduce frownlines and facial tension around the eyes. Using the balls of your thumbs or index fingers, apply pressure to either side of the top of your nose for a few seconds. Gradually work down to the nostrils, concentrating on the cartilage at the edge of your nose.

LIFT THE LID

Droopy eyes can be caused by weak muscle tone in the upper eyelid. Gently massage the surrounding area between your lids and your brows, and along your temples, for a few minutes once a day to improve muscle tone and circulation.

TAKE THE PINCH

Stimulate circulation in your facial skin by pinching the jawline. Start at the chin, pinching with your thumbs underneath and your fingers on top, and holding for ten seconds. Move along the lower jawbone until you reach the earlobes. Aim for four to five pinches to cover the area.

PAMPER YOUR PEEPERS

Reduce eye strain and wrinkles caused by squinting with a regenerating eye massage. Work fingers along the orbital bone around your eye sockets. Start at the outer edge and work backwards and forwards from the bridge of your nose at least three times.

GET IN CHEEKY CONDITION

Boost cheek tautness with a quick circulation-boosting massage. Work under the cheekbones with two fingers of each hand, pressing gently, from the middle of your face to the top of your ears, then work back to the middle.

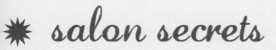

salon secrets

TIP YOUR THERAPIST

If you liked the therapy and want the same person next time, give them a 10% tip as you leave to show your appreciation. They'll find space in their schedule for you if you want another appointment!

DIP INTO THE DEAD SEA

You can buy these products for use at home, but the more powerful ingredients are reserved for salon formulations. The treatments use the mineral-rich mud from the Dead Sea to detoxify and revitalize skin.

BRAVE MICRODERMABRASION

This skin-booster uses aluminium oxide particles to slough off the outermost layers, leaving complexions brighter and evening out tone and colour. There are home-based alternatives, but professional is best to reduce redness and irritation post-treatment.

HARVEST YOUR OWN CELLS

An alternative to Botox that uses your own skin cells, Isolagen treatments takes a tiny skin cell sample from behind your ear. The cells are grown in a lab and re-injected into frown lines, crow's feet and wrinkly hands. They are used medically to heal scarring from burns. You are using your own, younger skin cells, preserved cryogenically, to rejuvenate your skin. Four or more treatments are needed to see the benefits.

BE ALERT TO ALLERGIES

If you're allergic to shellfish, tell your beauty therapist before beginning any treatments. Many face products and wraps contain ground shells or marine products, which could cause an allergic reaction, such as redness or swelling. As a matter of course, always warn the therapist about all allergies, sensitivities and medical conditions.

QUICK-TIME MAKEOVERS

If you are time-poor and need a quick makeover for a special event, book an express treatment. Many hair and beauty salons offer a cut and colour combined with body treatments, such as manicures, massages and brow shaping.

TIGHT AND FIRM

Thermage and Thermacool treatments work by heating the underlying tissues of the skin, causing the collagen to contract so your skin firms and wrinkles smooth out.

CACI YOUR ASSETS

CACI technology isn't just used for the face – it can also be used to create a nonsurgical "bust lift" by targeting sagging skin on the chest and firming the bust.

SMOOTH SPOTS WITH SMOOTHBEAM

A good salon choice for spotty or greasy skins, smoothbeam lasers are used to target oil glands, which slows down oil production, helping prevent spots and blackheads, and to stimulate collagen production, which can tighten pores.

FILL OUT WITH FAT TRANSFERS

Autolgous fat transplantation plumps up skin using your own fat that has been liposuctioned from your thighs or abdomen. This can be used for deep lines, lip augmentation and acne scars.

REMODEL WITH RADIO FREQUENCY

Skin tightening the jowly bits of the cheek that hang down below the jawline in ugly little bulges is now possible with a non-surgical procedure that involves radiofrequency remodelling. It contracts the skin that has stretched, giving it a lift and reducing the size of the jowls.

MASSAGE AWAY PUFFINESS

A great instant pick-me-up if you are suffering from puffy or problem skin is a manual lymphatic drainage (MLD) massage, which boosts circulation, detoxifies and reduces fluid build-up. It is used to improve cellulite and stretch marks, too.

BOOST YOUR OXYGEN

A fabulous salon treatment loved by models is a facial designed to boost the oxygen levels in your skin by pumping oxygen onto the face via a metal tube from a tank. It leaves a genuine (if short-lived) glow and skin feels rejuvenated. To stimulate the effect, try oxygen creams.

ASK FOR A JEWEL

Some skin conditions can respond to electronic gem therapy, which involves passing light rays through gemstones. For eczema sufferers, emeralds and sapphires are used to zap problem areas.

LIGHT UP YOUR LIFE

Salon treatments that involve an application of yellow light to reduce the bacterial count in skin can reduce acne by up to half after just one treatment. Called Light Therapy, it's a miracle for problem skin.

SALINE KISSES COMING SOON

Dermatologists are working on saline lip implants that will be inserted through tiny incisions along lip borders and then inflated with salt water, resulting in smooth but bigger lips.

THERMO-TARGET THREAD VEINS

Thermo-coagulation is a vein-removal technique based on a high-frequency wave producing a thermal lesion that reduces the vein. A very fine needle is inserted into the vein and it disappears instantaneously.

PIECE OF THE ACTION

GABA is a surface-applied ingredient that has been used pharmaceutically to freeze muscles, mimicking the effects of Botox without an invasive injection.

A NICE LITTLE LEARNER

If you're stuck in a rut, book a lesson with a top make-up artist. They can teach you professional tricks and introduce you to new colours and products. Boutiques and salons also have staff on hand for lessons but the smaller ones tend to be less hectic and more individualistic than those at big department stores.

SHARE IN A FLOTATION

Your bath is just too small for a flotation experience so a salon visit is a must. Excellent for toning and relaxing, flotation entails floating in darkness in a special tank. The treatment helps your body and mind relax in peace and harmony.

HANDLE HYLAFORM WITH CARE

Dermal injections involve plumping up facial lines and wrinkles by injecting small amounts of the filler into them. Hylaform uses hyaluronic acid, from rooster combs, as its key compound, which could cause allergic reactions. Non-animal derived hyaluronic is used in Restylane and Perlane.

PULSE AWAY PIGMENT

Pulsed light technology is an alternative to lasers. With this salon treatment, pulses of intense, concentrated light are directed onto the skin and absorbed by the melanin in pigmented lesions, such as age, sun and liver spots, which evens out pigmentation. The technique is also used for hair removal and blemishes.

HOT SUGAR BODY POLISH

Don't try this at home, unless you're prepared to caramelize yourself. A hot sugar solution is applied to the skin and all-over massage is used to stimulate circulation and make the skin glow.

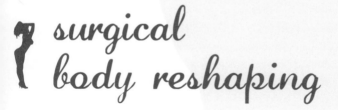

surgical body reshaping

RESIZE MY THIGHS

Losing weight may result in slack and saggy skin around your thighs that no amount of exercise will shift. Thigh-lift surgery is used to remove excess skin and fat from both the inside and the outside of the upper thigh, but the surgery will leave a noticeable scar around the groin.

NO MIRACLE CURE

Liposuction can remove fat from beneath the skin and remove fatty deposits, and if you regain weight afterwards it will mostly be in areas not suctioned. However, it cannot cure cellulite, tighten loose skin or take out fat from underneath muscles.

SLIM AND SEXY CALVES

Some types of liposuction use smaller suction tubes to suck out fat, which has revolutionized the results that can be achieved on delicate areas like calves and ankles. Lower leg shape is often determined by muscle tone and underlying skeleton, so the results are often quite subtle.

PERK UP SAGGY BREASTS

Excess weight and the passage of time can cause breasts to droop and lose their shape. Breast uplift surgery can be done without altering the size of your bosom, as the surgeon simply makes a small incision around the breast to reposition the nipple higher and remove excess skin from below.

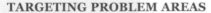

TARGETING PROBLEM AREAS

Liposuction targets certain areas of the body where hard to shift fatty
deposits have built up, like middle-aged tummies, hips and buttocks.
Up to 2.25–4.5 kg (5–10 lbs) of fat and fluids can be removed at one
time. For perfect results, skin needs to show some elasticity.

LOSE BREAST BULK

Breast reduction is a relatively simple operation for women who have
large, heavy breasts that cause them back and neck pain. Big breasts
that are out of proportion to your size can make dressing difficult, and
make you more self-conscious. An operation will leave you standing
tall with less upper body bulk and more confidence.

TINY TUCKS REDUCE BINGO WINGS

A hidden-scar arm lift (brachioplasty) removes excess skin and fat
from the upper arms. A tiny incision is made in the armpit, and fat
is removed from the upper arm while excess skin is pulled upwards
towards the underarm, leaving arms firm and toned.

LESS EXTREME THAN LIPOSUCTION

A fat-busting treatment that is safer and less invasive than liposuction
can suck fat from double chins as well as tighten up wobbly knees and
bingo wings. Known as SmartLipo, the procedure uses a fine laser
probe which is inserted into the skin in the problem area to increase
the temperature of the fat cells. This causes them to break down into
liquid, which the body is then able to expel.

BOTTOMS AND THIGHS

After losing a lot of weight, you may find that you have loose, sagging
skin around your buttocks and thighs, which no amount of exercise
and healthy living will remedy. An operation can be done to raise
and tighten the skin in these areas. If both thighs and buttocks are
operated on, the procedure is known as a lower body lift. Cuts will be
made in as unobtrusive a place as possible, and you will need to wear
a compression garment after the operation to reduce swelling and to
help to shrink and tighten the skin.

TUCK AWAY THAT TUMMY

A tummy tuck is not intended for weight control, but can be used for women who have excess skin and fat in their abdominal area, usually after substantial weight loss. An abdominoplasty requires the surgeon to make an incision across the bikini area, and then remove fat and skin; it will tighten the tummy muscles and leave the abdomen firmer and flatter.

SUPERSIZE ME

The type of breast implant – silicone or saline – plus the size and shape of your new breasts should all be carefully considered with your surgeon. The incision can be made under the arm where it is hidden, around the nipple, or under the breast. Full recovery time is about six weeks, and most implants have a lifetime guarantee.

GET PREPARED

If you decide on plastic surgery, it's very important to find a good surgeon and to talk through any issues beforehand. Be realistic too about what surgery can achieve – it won't hold back the clock for ever but it will help you to age at your preferred rate. Your surgeon can advise you on what to need to do to prepare yourself, such as losing weight, stopping smoking, cutting out alcohol and taking extra doses of vitamin C.

smooth & trim

BALANCE OUT BREASTS

If you have uneven breasts, don't worry – most women do. Try an enhanced bra with the enhancement taken out of the cup that holds the larger breast, or use one of those "chicken fillet" external implants.

LOOK LEAN BY GOING GREEN

Did you know that green tea can help you lose weight by stimulating your basal metabolic rate to help you burn calories more easily? Two cups a day is ample.

BRUSH AWAY BLEMISHES

Dry body brushing kickstarts the circulation and aids the elimination of toxins, which prevents skin looking puffy and helps you avoid blemishes, spots and dry patches, especially those white bumps that appear on the arms and legs that are a sign of congested skin.

STAND UP STRAIGHT

Improve your bust line simply by standing up straighter. Improved posture will naturally lift the ribcage and enable the breasts to sit more upright on the chest. Imagine a golden string through your spine, pulling your head upwards.

BRUSH AWAY BLEMISHES

Dry body brushing kickstarts the circulation and aids the elimination of toxins, which prevents skin looking puffy and helps you avoid blemishes, spots and dry patches, especially those white bumps that appear on the arms and legs that are a sign of congested skin.

STAND UP STRAIGHT

Improve your bust line simply by standing up straighter. Improved posture will naturally lift the ribcage and enable the breasts to sit more upright on the chest. Imagine a golden string through your spine, pulling your head upwards.

FIRM WITH A GEL

The delicate skin on the neck and upper chest is a target for sun damage and ages fast. In fact, you may notice the neck lines and crevices before you notice them on your face. The best formulas for this area are gel- or serum-based and not only deliver a sunscreen and anti-ageing moisturizer, but fade age spots and firm loose skin, albeit temporarily.

BUST TONERS

Toners formulated for tightening the bust area have an instant but temporary effect, though the ingredients they deliver have longterm benefits for skin health. Though there is no nonsurgical route to a bust lift, these treatments can assist in cell metabolism and strengthen and renew the skin to leave the texture refined. Massage in gently, avoiding the nipples.

TAKE UP ARMS

Regular massage will help prevent rough skin and pimples on the arms. Massage in almond or olive oil to boost circulation and concentrate on the back of arms, where fat deposits can cause uneven skin.

ALL FOR ALMOND OIL

Use sweet almond oil after a bath or shower to coat the body in the vitamin A-rich oil, which the skin will absorb where it needs it. An excellent, penetrating emollient, it is useful for all skin types and relieves itching and irritation. Concentrate particularly on dry areas and, if possible, leave on overnight.

GRAB A GRAPEFRUIT

Grapefruit is an excellent choice for a healthy fruit that will make you look good. It is a natural diuretic, which prevents bloating and water retention, and helps you stay slim. Choose it as a healthy starter or a mid-afternoon snack. Many beauty products contain grapefruit purely for its reinvigorating scent.

GET SLICK WITH LOTION

To give yourself an extra watery boost and lock in extra moisture, slather on moisturizing creams directly after a bath or shower while your skin is still damp. Body creams and lotions that contain gentle chemical exfoliators, including glycolic acid and salicylic acid can help even out skin tone, while "contouring" or "lifting" creams will improve skin texture.

BEAT THE BLOAT

Stock up your diet with natural diuretics. Watercress, watermelon, fennel and peppermint tea can all stop your body bloating and retaining water, which can make eyes and cheeks look puffy – as well as your tummy – and add pounds.

MASSAGE AS YOU MOISTURIZE

When you apply a body oil or lotion, do so using massage techniques: use sweeping, upward motions towards your heart to give your lymphatic drainage a boost. Taking time to really work the oil into your skin will help it penetrate and imbue a lustrous glow.

sun safety & tanning

PROTECT WITH PLE

If you are concerned about the effects of sun damage on the skin, consider taking an oral supplement that offers photo-protection, such as polypodium leucotomas extract, or PLE. Recent clinical research has found that this extract from a South American fern has powerful antioxidant and photoprotective properties. Native Americans have been using it to treat inflammatory disorders and skin diseases for centuries.

THE TAN WON'T LAST

As you age, the pigment in your skin is less active, with the result that your skin will tan less easily with time. Take notice of this simple fact to ensure you don't accidentally stay out in the sun longer than safe limits. If you like the look of a tan, rely on self-tanning products which will be more effective than your own body's pigment-making capabilities.

HANDS OFF

Sun damage affects all of your body, not just the face. Always remember to cover your hands with an SPF 20 when you spend time in the sun to avoid photo-ageing wrinkles and liver spots, the telltale signs of ageing.

A SAFE TAN

When our skin turns brown it has been burnt, and damaged cells will always contain some residual changes that stay in our DNA and which may over time result in cancerous cells. The only safe tan is a fake one, where the active ingredient DHA reacts with proteins in our skin to stain it and make it darker in colour.

STAY YOUNG WITHOUT SUN

Exposure to sunlight leads to premature skin ageing and the cumulative effects of wrinkling, blotchy pigmentation and roughness. Sun-damaged skin is easier to bruise and is less elastic.

USE SPF 30 EVERY DAY

To avoid the damage the sun can do to your skin, it is essential to limit the time you expose your body to direct sunlight. You should always cover up your face with a sunscreen that has at least an SPF 30 and five-star UVA protection. Get into the habit of applying a sunscreen every day.

SLAP IT ON

Most people apply suncream to their face and body at the start of the day and forget about it. During a typical two-week beach holiday, when you are exposed to sun on a daily basis, you should expect to get through two 250 ml (8 fl oz) bottles of sun protection, so keep slapping it on all over throughout the day.

SUN SAFETY FOR DARK SKINS

All skin needs protecting from harmful UVA and UVB rays, and while pale skin must use a higher SPF, even people with dark skin should never use anything lower than an SPF 15.

DON'T DO SUNBEDS

Although a sunbed does not expose the body to UVB rays (the ones that affect the outer layers of the skin and cause sun damage) it can still cause burning and premature ageing because the intensity of the UVA rays is so strong.

SHADES AND HAT COMPULSORY

Strong sunlight can damage eyes, and particularly the fine skin around the eyes. Keep covered up throughout the day with sunglasses and a broad-brimmed hat to protect the face and hair.

TAKE COVER AT THE HOTTEST TIME

Never spend more than four hours a day lying out in the sun, and take cover inside during the hottest hours of the day between 12 pm and 3 pm when the sun is at its most powerful and exposure of the skin should be avoided. Hair and eyes can also be damaged, so cover up with a broad-brimmed hat and sunglasses.

WINTER PROTECTION

Although we often remember to protect ourselves from the sun in summer, it is equally important throughout the year. Always wear a moisturizer with an SPF and sunglasses when the winter sun appears, especially if you are out in the snow, which reflects the light.

CLOUDY DAY DAMAGE

Don't make the mistake of thinking your skin is safe from sun damage when the weather is overcast. Up to 80% of UV light can pass though cloud cover, so you still need protection on grey days and when sitting under a beach umbrella. Wear a daily moisturizer with SPF even when the sky is cloudy.

GLOBAL WARMING

If you want to avoid ageing liver spots and sun damage you should be wearing an antioxidant moisturizer that contains a sunscreen all year round. Look for one that contains zinc oxide and titanium dioxide to block the sun.

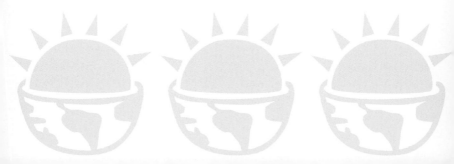

LEG CHECK

The most common place to develop a malignant melanoma is on your legs, so make sure you check them regularly for freckles or moles that have changed shape or are seeping blood. Don't be tempted to sunbathe without sun protection on your legs.

GET PREPARED

Don't wait until you are out in the sun to apply a protective lotion to your skin. Sunscreen needs time to work so smooth it on about 20 minutes before you go outside, and don't be stingy with it – use liberal amounts.

DIFFERENT NEEDS

Your face and body require different products to protect them from sun damage. Always use SPF 30 on your face and at least an SPF 15 on your body, and make sure that your lotion has a high UVA filter.

GREY DAY PROTECTION

A good day moisturizer not only kickstarts circulation after the nocturnal shutdown, but also helps to fight the damaging effects of the sun even in winter and on grey days.

PREP UP FOR GOOD TAN

A fake tan can even out the complexion and disguise dark circles and broken veins but won't work unless it's correctly applied. Thorough exfoliation of the skin is crucial for a good fake tan. Do it at home or get the therapist to do it before your treatment, followed by generous moisturizing to ensure colour goes on smoothly and there are no streaky stripes.

GENETIC TESTING

One cancer expert has developed a skin test called the Skinphysical, which can read the sun damage in your DNA. The results determine how much damage has already occurred and how to maximize your protection in future years. See www.skinphysical.co.uk

SUN-SENSITIVE PERFUME

Avoid wearing fragrance that contains alcohol when sunbathing as it makes skin photosensitive, and can result in dryness, burning and pigmentation. The eau de toilette version of your favourite perfume will usually have a lower alcohol content.

CHOOSE COLOURED SELF-TAN

The best self-tanners are those that are bronzed and instantly deposit a layer of non-permanent colour on the skin so you can see if you have missed any spots.

DON'T SWALLOW IT

The chemical DHA (dihydroxyacetone in spray-on tanners) is approved for external application only. Put cotton wool in your nostrils and keep your mouth closed during application in a tanning booth.

TAN FOR HEALTHY-LOOKING HANDS

Hands are one of the areas that show the most signs of ageing but they can look a lot better with a little light-coloured self-tan. This can be a tricky area to work on, so use your fingertips to lightly stroke and blend well, then use a facial wipe to clean the palms.

MAINTAINING THAT TAN

After a fake tan use a light all-over body moisturizer to avoid flakiness. Take quick showers with minimal soaping (as opposed to luxurious bubble baths) and avoid heavy exercise, because sweat will dissipate the tan, leaving you covered in uneven patches.

AIRBRUSH TAN IN A CAN

If you don't have the time (or money) for a trip to the salon you can now buy a facial tanning spray in a can. With micro-fine particles you can expect to see professional results for a fraction of the cost, and not a patchy streak in sight.

THROW ON THE TOWEL

If you burn the skin on your face, place a damp, cold flannel over the burnt area for ten minutes to take away redness and swelling. Avoid alcohol, smoke and further sun until the redness fades, and use aftersun moisturizer twice a day.

HEAD FOR A SCREEN TEST

Don't be tempted to use intensive moisturizers or conditioners in your hair in the hope that they'll keep your locks protected in the sun – the sun burns them up, which can make hair even drier. Instead, use a hair-specific sunscreen for ultimate protection.

BE A SHADY LADY

Take care of the delicate skin around the eyes with a pair of polarized sunglasses. Wraparound styles that fully cover the whole eye area and the sides of the face are best, as they protect the skin prone to crow's feet and fine under-eye lines.

KEEP CREAM COOL

Sun cream is more effective when it's kept cool, so make sure you leave it in the shade if you're on the beach, or the sun's heat could denature the active ingredients and make it less effective.

DON'T GO FOR THE BURN

Not only is burnt skin dangerous, it will peel faster, leaving you with pink patches and a dry, flaky surface. Use suntan lotions and creams with added moisturizers and pace yourself with sun exposure for a smooth, even tan.

LET'S GET THIS CLEAR

For beautiful beach skin, go for the model's choice – a clear or yellow-tinged sunscreen with a high factor instead of the white lotions that make your skin appear pale and pasty. These varieties will give your skin a golden appearance while delivering high protection at the same time. Sprays are best for even coverage.

GET PHYSICAL

If you have sensitive skin, allergies or acne, opt for a physical sunscreen that contains mineral ingredients to block out the rays rather than a chemical-based version containing parabens, which have been shown to increase skin sensitivity.

DO THE DOSE RIGHT

For a sunscreen to live up to its SPF rating, 2 mg should be applied for every square centimetre (½ inch) of exposed skin, which means on average you should be using 100 mg for every four whole-body applications. Most people don't use anything like enough.

TAN WITH TANGERINES

Antioxidant vitamins A, C and E – found in red, yellow and orange fruit and vegetables – can help limit damage to skin from the sun's rays by mopping up damaging free radicals in the body.

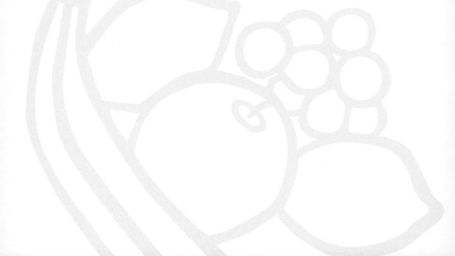

PUCKER UP

Don't forget lips need sun protection too – the skin on them is thinner than anywhere else on your face, and overexposure to the sun and elements can leave them dry and coarse. Use a sunscreen specially formulated for the lips with a minimum of SPF 15.

MAKE-UP IF YOU MUST

If you really can't brave the beach without make-up, apply waterproof cosmetics first and then pat sunblock over the top to ensure even protection and to prevent make-up from sliding down your face. Avoid full foundation, opting instead for a touch of concealer. Consider having your eyelashes and brows (if pale) tinted to keep your features from looking faded in the sun.

JOIN THE BAND

Worried about sun damage? Invest in a UV wristband, a disposable band you wear on your wrist that measures sun exposure and changes colour when you've had enough.

BE AN A-LIST STAR

It's not just your suncream's UVB-protective SPF rating that counts – make sure your cream's got a UVA-blocking star rating as well. It goes from one to five, with five being the strongest.

COOL DOWN SUMMER BURN

Chlorine, sun and high temperatures can make the skin on your legs more prone to post-shave stinging and rashes. Use a lotion with aloe vera to soothe – studies have shown that aloe vera improves the skin's ability to hydrate itself and that it speeds healing. Store the lotion in the fridge for 20 minutes before application for a soothing treat that will really cool skin.

HANDS OFF THE TAN!

Prevent tell-tale orange palms by applying a tiny amount of silicone-based "frizz-control" hair product to your palms, which blocks the pigment from absorbing into your skin.

WITCH WAY TO STOP THE ITCH?

Ease sunburnt areas and prevent itching, soreness and further damage with a homemade body lotion. Mix 120 ml (4 fl oz) of witch hazel with 60 ml (2 fl oz) each of aloe vera gel, baby oil and high-factor sunscreen.

FAKE IT FLAWLESSLY

When you're choosing a fake tan lotion, look for one that contains erythrulose, a unique DHA enhancer. The combination of DHA and erythrulose helps ensure a more even, streakless, longlasting tan without increasing dryness.

STOP THE FADE

Keep your fake tan looking great all week by avoiding moisturizers that contain any of the following: Retin-A, AHAs, BHAs or glycolic acids. These ingredients will slough off the dead cells in the top layer of the skin and make your tan fade faster.

SPRAY-ON SUN

Modern airbrush spray-tanning booths will give you an all-over aloe-based DHA tan without your body ever seeing the sun. One session will last about a week and you can choose from a range of shades. A good idea to ease yourself from a tan into a wintry pallor is to invest in a series of sessions – a once-a-week session will keep your tan going for months to come.

EXFOLIATE DAILY

Prepare your skin for self-tanning by exfoliating daily for the three or four days before you apply it and using moisturizer liberally following exfoliation to build up smoothness and hydration in the skin and prevent uneven streaks.

HIDE THE TIDE MARK

If tan lines caused by bikinis, tops, shorts and socks are blighting your quest for the all-over tan, smooth out marks by applying small amounts of fake tan (mixed with moisturizer at first so you don't go too dark) to give yourself an even-looking tan. Simply reapply as the tan fades.

FAKE TANNING FOR BLONDES

After applying fake tan to the face, sweep a tissue around the hairline and over the brows to avoid colouring light hair. Don't forget to scrub the nails and palms of the hands afterwards, too.

HAVE A CLOSE SHAVE

Shaving not only removes hairs, it also serves to exfoliate the skin by stretching off the top layer, so it's a great choice the day before you apply self-tan. But avoid shaving for a day or two afterwards as it could weaken the tan.

DRY SKIN MAY GO DARK

Dry skin around knees, elbows and ankles picks up self-tan colour more, leading to dark patches. Instead of applying tan neat, mix it with moisturizer for these areas.

MOISTURIZE MODERATELY

Too much moisturizer is one of the biggest fake tan mistakes – it creates a barrier between the skin and the tan, making the tanning dye less effective and more prone to slipping and streaks. Wait until the body cream has soaked in before applying fake tan.

BUILD UP TO SUCCESS

Perfect the no-streaks, natural-looking tan with a little patience! Instead of slathering it all on at once, apply a light layer of self-tan at a time and build up the colour with a second application a few days later.

Natural Beauty

IT IS OFTEN SAID THAT beauty starts from the inside out, and it is certainly true that good nutrition can make a big difference to the health of your skin, eyes and hair. From superfoods to vitamin-packed health-boosters, this chaper targets beauty concerns from a nutritional point of view. Natural remedies for beauty problems as well as homemade and all-natural "green" treatments are included, as are ethical beauty concerns such as buying fairtrade and harmful ingredients in beauty products.

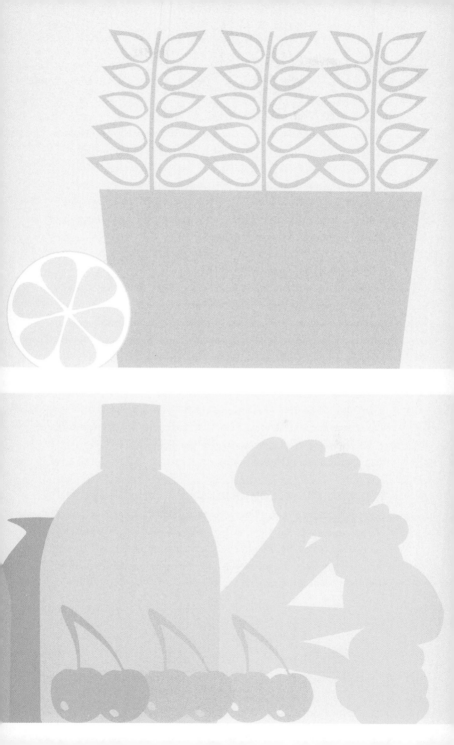

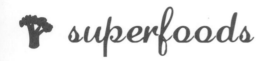 **superfoods**

CHECK OUT ORAC FOODS

Oxygen Radical Absorbance Capacity (ORAC) is an American test tube analysis that has pinpointed the highest levels of antioxidants in fruit and vegetables. Early findings by the US Department of Agriculture suggest ORAC foods may help slow the ageing process in the brain as well as the body, and young and middle-aged people may be able to reduce risk of diseases of ageing, including senility, by adding high-ORAC foods to their diets.

TOP-SCORING ORAC FOODS

The high levels of antioxidants found in the ORAC foods (see above) come from plant pigments called polyphenols, and it is thought to be the combination of vitamins, iron and folic acid that makes them so effective. Top-scoring ORAC foods are avocado, blueberries, broccoli, garlic, kale, plums, raisins, red grapes and spinach.

BE AN OLD PRUNE

Dried plums – prunes – have been given the ultimate superfood status, as they are thought to contain the highest level of antioxidants, which neutralize the dangerous free radicals associated with DNA degradation and accelerated ageing.

CHEER UP WITH CHERRIES

For a quick burst of something sweet that will give you instant energy and raise blood sugar levels slowly, eat cherries. They contain antioxidants called flavonoids, which have been reported to have antiviral, anti-allergic, antiplatelet, anti-inflammatory, antitumour and antioxidant activities.

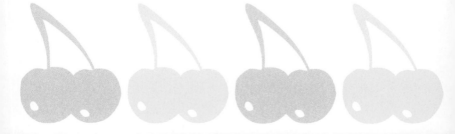

LOOK FOR NUTRACEUTICALS

Wise up to "functional foods" that have specific health benefits because they have had health-boosting extras added to them, like margarine spread that has plant sterols to help lower cholesterol, or water with added calcium.

A-STAR

The most useful of vitamins for healthy skin, vitamin A has the ability to calm red and blotchy skin and is also thought to visibly reduce lines and wrinkles.

SPECIFIC HEALTH BOOSTERS

Purple anthocyanins that are found in blueberries are known to strengthen tiny blood vessels and so help reduce spider veins and the flushed red appearance of rosacea.

FULL-FAT SKINCARE

A diet that is devoid of all fats will deprive your skin of the essential fatty acids it needs, and leave your skin looking dry and dull. Essential Fatty Acids (EFAs) are absolutely vital for good health as they help lower cholesterol and keep hair and skin healthy. They can't be made in your body so they must be supplied through your diet. Nuts, avocado and oily fish are all good sources.

SARDINES FOR SUPPER

It is recommended that women eat two portions of oily fish a week and sardines provide an easy way to achieve this – served on toast they make a perfect early-evening snack. High in omega-3 fatty acids, they provide some of the best protection against heart disease and strokes, and help to keep skin soft, supple and young-looking.

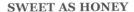
SWEET AS HONEY

Renowned for its medicinal properties since the time of the ancient Egyptians, dark-coloured honeys such as buckwheat possess more antioxidants than the lighter varieties, and also provide nutrients for the growth of new tissue, helping skin rejuvenate itself and stay young-looking.

EAT YOUR GREENS

Learn to love green foods like cabbage, leeks and broccoli, which are rich in sulphur, the "beauty mineral" that promotes healthy skin and nails. They also contain high levels of antioxidants, which help to prevent skin from ageing.

BUSH BENEFITS

Try redbush tea instead of the traditional cuppa. A herbal brew drunk for centuries by the San of southern Africa, its taste is similar to ordinary tea. It's also caffeine-free and packed with antioxidants.

GOJI GOOD FOR CELLULITE

One leading skincare expert has dubbed goji juice the "cellulite assassin". This energy-boosting drink contains more betacarotene than carrots and more iron than spinach.

ONE AMAZING LITTLE BERRY

Known as one of the anti-ageing super foods, the acai berry is indigenous to the Amazon rainforests, and contains the same compounds called anthocyanins that makes red wine good for us. Try concentrated fruit drinks, or eat the berry itself, to help slow down the ageing process.

SEARCH OUT SELENIUM

This is a very important antioxidant that works with vitamin E to prohibit free-radical damage to the cell membrane. It is also thought to help prevent cancer, protect against heart and circulatory diseases and promote healthy eyes, skin and hair. Good natural sources include Brazil nuts, kidney, liver and wholemeal bread.

NUTTY ABOUT NUTS

Unsalted nuts make a great snack as they are full of EFAs, which can't be manufactured by the body and which are needed to speed up the digestive system and keep skin moist and fresh-looking. Stick to a small handful as they are highly calorific.

CHEW UP ON ALMOND SKINS

Research has shown that almond skins alone contain 20 potent antioxidants to protect against heart disease. They are also rich in vitamin E which is thought to help slow down the ageing process.

ENERGY-BOOSTING BERRY

Freshly juiced blackcurrants contain a host of antioxidants that can protect cells from premature ageing, as well as lower cholesterol levels and guard against cancer.

SHOT OF WHEATGRASS

It may taste unusual, but a small glass of wheatgrass is packed with many essential minerals including calcium, magnesium, potassium, iron and sodium as well as vitamins A, B C and E, all of which are needed for healthy teeth, hair and skin. It's very easy to grow your own.

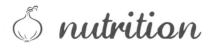

nutrition

STRENGTHENING SULPHUR

Asparagus is rich in sulphur, a mineral that's vital for strong nails as it strengthens the nail bed. Other sources include seafood, onion, garlic and cabbage.

BEAT CELLULITE WITH SAGE

Sage is known for its cellulite-busting properties so try to incorporate plenty of the fresh herb into your diet. It works by improving the digestion and breaking down the fatty deposits in the body which cause cellulite.

POPEYE POWER

There's no point spending money on manicures if your nails are weak and brittle. Spinach is rich in essential B vitamins, which are important for helping nails to grow stronger. Eat raw in salads or lightly steamed.

STRONG COLOURS COUNT MORE

All fresh fruit and vegetables contain powerful antioxidants but in general the deeper and more intense the colour, the higher the content. Choose red and orange pepper, tomatoes, cranberries, pomegranates and broccoli.

BEANS FOR A BEAUTIFUL BOB

Some experts believe that an overload of toxins in the body leads to dull hair. So flush out your system on the cheap by eating plenty of fibre-rich foods such as lentils, beans and wholegrain cereals.

BROCCOLI BOOSTER

This super-veg has as many nutrients as lots of expensive multivitamins. Broccoli is a good source of vitamin A, which helps reduce oil production; vitamin K, which reduces the formation of bruises; and vitamin C, which is a powerful antioxidant that prevents fine lines and wrinkles.

POLISH WITH PORRIDGE

For a morning glow, breakfast on porridge with skimmed milk, topped with flaxseeds and blueberries and a glass of orange juice – all the best ingredients for healthy skin.

SCAR SOLUTION

Beauty products designed to aid healing are very expensive. Eating plenty of vitamin C-rich fruit can help scars heal more quickly. Good sources include citrus fruits such as lemon, orange and grapefruit, but the richest source is kiwi fruit. Just one kiwi fruit has twice the vitamin C content of an orange.

SILKY SILICA

Silica is a mineral that is important for keeping your hair elastic, shiny and healthy. It can be found in oats, cucumber skin, onions and bean sprouts, which means a healthy and economical diet of porridge (oatmeal) for breakfast and salad for lunch.

BOOST WITH BIOTIN

Biotin is another building block for healthy nails. So dump the expensive perfect-nail pills and tuck into biotin-rich foods like eggs, soya and cauliflower. A diet rich in biotin is guaranteed to help strengthen and thicken your nails.

DRINK GREEN TEA

Favoured by celebrities including Sophie Dahl and Victoria Beckham, green tea has a number of beauty benefits. It is naturally rich in antioxidants, which help to protect against free radicals and premature ageing. The leaves can also be used as a gentle exfoliant to give your skin a healthy glow.

BOOST YOUR BEAUTY WITH NATURAL YOGURT

Yogurt has many benefits for natural beauty, both internally and externally. Live yogurt contains bacteria, which benefits the digestive system and helps to keep skin clear. It is also an ideal ingredient for a homemade face pack due to its natural exfoliating properties.

SCOFF FRUIT

Fruit is essential for healthy skin, not only because of all the vitamins and minerals, but also because it contains high levels of water, which also serve to keep skin hydrated. Pimples or congested skin in the forehead area are often a sign of constipation or blockage in the lymphatic systems, which can be relieved by eating plenty of fruit and vegetables.

MIX UP A BEAUTY SNACK

Fix yourself a mini-meal of low-fat muesli mixed with ground flaxseeds and dried fruit, topped with plain yogurt. For another beauty-boosting snack, drink tomato juice with a splash of lemon.

GO FOR GRAPEFRUIT

Eat well for gorgeous-looking skin, by fixing yourself a lunch of grilled shrimp salad with grapefruit and watercress. These ingredients contain high levels of zinc and antioxidants to boost skin healing. Top it with parsley, which is rich in vitamin A, chlorophyll, vitamin B12, folic acid, vitamin C and iron – all good for skin health.

CUT SUGAR FOR CLEAR SKIN

Sugar, refined carbohydrates and saturated fats can contribute to blemishes. If you think your diet is to blame, try a gentle detox programme to purify your system.

EAT STRAWBERRIES

High in antioxidants, strawberries can be beneficial in the fight against premature ageing and wrinkles. They are particularly high in vitamin C, which is important for the formation of collagen – a key element that helps to keep skin firm. Strawberries also help to protect against broken capillaries beneath the skin's surface.

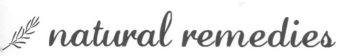# natural remedies

HYDRATE WITH FRUITS AND NUTS

For extra-dry, scaly or flaky skin, look for products that contain sweet almond oil, apricot and berries like blackberry, all of which pack a super-hydrating punch and will help regenerate tissues without blocking pores.

DETOX TWICE A YEAR

One way to get clearer eyes and a radiant glow is to detoxify. Natural health experts recommend detoxing twice a year – around spring and autumn – to give your skin and overall health a boost. Ridding your body of everyday toxins can help to improve the texture and appearance of your skin and hair.

COME TO THE OIL

Essential oils are relaxing, detoxifying and nourishing. They are absorbed very easily and won't leave your face shiny. Rose oil is particularly noted for its soothing properties and restores suppleness to mature skins – blend a few drops with patchouli and geranium oils in a carrier oil and apply a small amount nightly.

PASS THE PARSLEY JUICE

Natural parsley juice (or parsley infusion) mixed with equal amounts of lemon juice, orange juice and redcurrant juice can be applied under your favourite face cream to keep freckles and other pigment spots less visible – the vitamin C in parsley regulates melanin production and evens skin tone. An infusion of fresh parsley can also be used to cleanse the skin to help clear acne.

EMBRACE GREASY HAIR

Give dry hair a natural conditioning treatment with olive oil. The oil helps repair split ends and improves the texture and appearance of parched hair. Heat the oil first in a cup placed in a pan of hot water. Then massage it into your hair and scalp and cover with a shower or swimming cap. Leave for 30 minutes before washing out with a gentle shampoo. Try this treatment once a week to give hair a natural boost or to remedy a dry, itchy scalp.

USE NATURAL HAIR DYES

Mainstream hair dyes use strong chemicals such as ammonia and have been linked to health problems including scalp irritation, facial swelling and even cancer. Choose natural dyes made with vegetable ingredients instead. These are still able to lighten hair by a couple of shades but without the potential side effects caused by harsher dyes and bleaches.

THE THYME IS RIGHT

Thyme contains deep-cleansing elements that remove dirt and debris in the skin. It also kills bacteria, which can cause acne, so an infusion is perfect for cleansing problem skin.

EMULATE AN EMU FOR SHINY HAIR

Emu oil is rich in omega-3 oils, which make your hair shiny and healthy. It is available in supplement or oil form, which you apply as a mask or conditioner.

CLEANSE WITH CARING OILS

Rather than invest in expensive creams, try a simple, natural cleanser, particularly good for mature skins. Apply a light film of almond or wheatgerm oil over your face, leave for a minute then remove with a warm, damp cloth or natural sponge.

HOME IN ON HOMEOPATHY

Homeopathic urtica tablets are derived from the stinging nettle, which not only has calming properties but also contains antihistamines, which naturally reduce the effects of allergic reactions.

GET EVEN WITH PRIMROSE

Many natural cosmetics include evening primrose oil as one of their key components. The oil has a high concentration of omega-3 oils and gamma-linolenic acid (GLA) that have been shown to help prevent and ease symptoms of psoriasis, eczema and other skin conditions. It also helps maintain the skin's water barrier. The essential fatty acids keep nails healthy and prevent cracks, and nourish the scalp and hair.

ALMOND EYES

Almond oil is a super all-round moisturizer. Use it on your lips and around your mouth, as a hand moisturizer or as a gentle eye make-up remover to smooth away wrinkles.

END ITCHING WITH ALOE

For those suffering extreme dryness or eczema, creams containing high levels of lavender and aloe vera can stop the itching. These ingredients have fast-acting, skin-soothing properties.

NATURAL WAYS TO COMBAT HAIR LOSS

Increasing the amount of protein-rich foods such as eggs, fish and tofu is one way to combat hair loss. Another is to take regular exercise, which will help boost circulation and increase blood flow to the scalp. Massaging your scalp also encourages the blood supply to stimulate hair growth.

JOJOBA FOR HAIR DRYNESS

Jojoba oil is waxy and rich in antioxidants; it will condition and nourish the hair shaft, leaving hair moisturized, smooth and sleek. Leave on overnight for a deep treatment, shampooing it out in the morning, or look for conditioner that contains it. Although plant-derived, jojoba is closer in make-up to sebum than to traditional vegetable oils.

BOOST SKIN HEALTH WITH APRICOTS

Apricots are a rich source of betacarotene, folic acid and iron, all of which boost skin health and help combat damaging free radicals and toxins from the environment and additives in food and cosmetics. The vitamin A helps keep skin soft and supple, and repairs skin cells and tissues.

PRESS AWAY PROBLEMS

In acupuncture, the area above your kneecap (measure the length of your kneecap and move exactly this distance above it and 2.5cm (1in) towards your inner thigh) is linked to skin problems. Press on each leg at the spot for at least a minute to reduce itching and inflammation of the skin.

SEARCH FOR WHITE BIRCH

White birch contains powerful lightening ingredients in the bark, which have been shown to work equally well on the skin. Used regularly, white birch can reduce areas of pigmentation and help make skin appear more even in colour.

COOL AS A CUCUMBER

Cucumber juice is good for blemishes because it refreshes and keeps skin hydrated without drying. It has mild astringent qualities that can help reduce redness and swelling, which makes spots look worse.

OVERCOME ITCHING WITH OATS

Oats contain natural anti-inflammatory properties which can help reduce skin flare-ups. For a simple home remedy, add a few cups of oats to a warm bath and wallow for 15 minutes to calm problem skin.

EASE ECZEMA WITH LINOLEIC ACID

Linoleic acid, found in many supplements and most nuts and seeds, is a powerful omega-6 oil, which helps eczema sufferers more than olive or fish oils.

CHOOSE THE GREY HAIR HERB

Fo ti, also known as the "grey hair herb", is claimed to darken and reduce the appearance of grey hair with regular use. It is available as a supplement, oil or ingredient in hair products.

SLEEP WELL WITH SANDALWOOD

As well as being an excellent moisturizer, a few drops of sandalwood oil in your bath can help decrease tension and relieve insomnia. Traditionally, it is also a natural antidepressant.

SALT OF THE EARTH

Salt baths encourage gentle detoxification of your whole body, and are particularly good for problem skin and fluid retention. Taken at the end of the day, they can also reduce tension and promote a good night's sleep.

IN THE PINK WITH ZINC

Zinc, which can be taken as a supplement or found in foods such as red meat, shellfish, sunflower seeds and peanuts, can help you keep skin clear and spot-free by boosting circulation and toxin removal.

TEA TREE WORKS A TREAT

Lavender and tea tree oil, as well as witch hazel, have natural antiseptic properties that can help prevent spots and bites becoming infected. Manuka honey is also a natural antiseptic, though it's a lot stickier!

SIP CAMOMILE FOR BEAUTIFUL EYES

Drinking camomile tea before bed is a good way to reduce under-eye bags, both by helping you get your beauty sleep and by reducing facial tension, which can cause dark circles to form.

SUPPLEMENT YOUR REGIME

There is a wide range of vitamin and mineral supplements available specifically to boost hair, skin and nails. Combination formulas, such as Viridian's Beauty Complex, provide a one-stop shop for women wanting to boost their general appearance. Individual supplements can be taken for specific areas, such as silica for hair and nails and omega-3 fatty acids for skin.

ROSEHIP OIL FOR MATURE SKINS

Although no beauty product can ward off the signs of ageing, mature skin benefits from rosehip oil. This plant oil contains nutrients to keep skin soft and supple. It is also extremely beneficial for people with scars or stretchmarks and will help to reduce their appearance. However, make sure it has been ethically sourced.

AVOID HARSH EYE WASHES

Eye-wash solutions often contain harsh chemicals. Brighten eyes naturally by using a cold-water wash instead. Then place a hot flannel over closed eyelids and press gently with your fingertips. Alternate this process several times and finish by placing a slice of chilled cucumber over each eye.

EAT STRAWBERRIES FOR WHITE TEETH

For centuries strawberries have been used to treat discoloured teeth. They can be mashed and applied directly onto teeth to help remove stains caused by red wine or tobacco, providing a healthy natural alternative to chemical teeth-whitening kits that can contain peroxide and titanium dioxide.

homemade treatments

SOOTHE SKIN WITH ALMONDS

Almond oil and ground almonds mixed with water are excellent ways to treat problem skin because of their gentle soothing properties, calming irritated nerve endings and reducing spotty outbreaks.

CAST YOUR OATS

Rather than spend money on expensive exfoliants, grab some oats from your kitchen cupboard. Crush them into a paste with some water and rub lightly over the face and neck for natural exfoliation and a healthy glow. Do not use on sensitive skins.

CRANBERRY DIY LIPSTICK

Avoid the petrochemicals and other ingredients found in lipsticks such as castor oil and even lead by making your own. Mix almond oil with ten fresh cranberries and a teaspoon of honey. Heat in a microwave for a couple of minutes. Mash the berries and then strain through a fine sieve before allowing it to cool.

PUT ON THE PARSLEY

Parsley is a great natural remedy for spots and blackheads because of its circulation-boosting properties. Grind the fresh herbs into a pulp and use as a face mask. Leave on for 10–15 minutes before rinsing off.

CURE SPOTS WITH FENUGREEK

Fenugreek leaves infused in a small amount of water and made into a paste can be used to target pimples, blackheads and dryness if applied and left overnight. Wash off with warm water in the morning.

GET A FACELIFT WITH EGG WHITE

Egg whites can be used to give an instant, natural facelift. Dab the whites directly onto lined areas and allow to dry before continuing your usual beauty routine. This gives skin an instant lift and helps to reduce the appearance of wrinkles. Egg whites can also be combined with honey and lemon juice for a reviving face pack.

FRESHEN UP WITH FENNEL

Chew on fennel seeds between meals instead of using conventional mouthwashes or toothpastes. The seeds have an anise-like flavour and act as an instant, natural breath freshener. If you choose organic seeds you will ensure that you're not coming into contact with any pesticide residues.

BICARBONATE OF SODA

Bicarbonate of soda (baking soda) is a very versatile natural ingredient. As well as being good for household cleaning, it can also be used for a number of different beauty treatments. Try mixing a small amount with your normal face-cleansing lotion for a home-made exfoliator. Using homemade treatments cuts down on the manufacture, packaging and expense of products, and so reduces your carbon footprint.

SOLVE PROBLEM AREAS WITH LEMON

Dry and discoloured skin on knees and elbows can be dealt with by using a fresh lemon. Cut it in half and sprinkle with a teaspoon of sugar, then rub the lemon halves into elbows and knees for a few minutes.

GO BARE

Instead of using nail polish, protect your nails by rubbing organic almond oil into the nails and cuticles to strengthen them. Clean discoloured nails by scrubbing them with a slice of lemon, which will get rid of stains, and gently buff for all-natural shine.

GIVE YOUR HAIR A DRINK

Lacklustre hair can be given a boost with beer. Mix up one part beer to three parts water and pour over your hair for the final rinse. The natural sugars in the beer will leave your hair smooth and shiny.

NOURISH SKIN WITH AVOCADO

Avocado is arguably the most important food for well-nourished skin. It provides essential fats necessary to prevent wrinkles and dryness. Incorporate avocado into your diet on a regular basis and apply it, mixed with natural yogurt, once a week as a face pack to get the benefits, internally and externally.

COFFEE GETS RID OF CELLULITE

Used coffee grounds can be used as a body exfoliator to get rid of cellulite. Take the used grounds from your morning coffee and rub them onto problem areas such as thighs during your shower for a natural cellulite treatment.

MAKE YOUR OWN BATH SALTS

Avoid fragrances and preservatives found in conventional bubble baths and create your own natural bath salts. A good recipe for a tension-relieving bath is to mix Epsom salts with baking soda and a few drops of lavender and marjoram essential oils.

MAKE YOUR OWN SOAPS

It is not that difficult to create your own homemade soaps and they will be gentler for skin than industrial versions. You will also know exactly what ingredients went into the product. Soap-making kits, widely available from craft stores and online shops, can be used successfully in the average kitchen. The main ingredients are vegetable oils, caustic soda and essential oils for fragrance.

CREATE YOUR OWN MAKE-UP REMOVER

Avoid chemical-based products and create your own make-up remover using milk. Dip an (organic) cotton wool ball into cold milk and use immediately. An alternative for oil-based make-up remover is sweet almond oil – look out for an organic variety if possible.

MAKE YOUR OWN BATH LOTIONS

Dried thyme and some raw oats make a relaxing and soothing all-natural herbal bath. Place them in a cheesecloth square and either tie it under the tap (faucet) as the water is running or place it directly in the bath. The oatmeal will soften the water.

MOISTURIZE WITH OLIVE OIL

For dry skin use olive oil, organic if possible. It has excellent moisturizing properties and has been traditionally used as an intensive conditioning and moisturizing treatment for areas prone to dry skin such as elbows, knees and feet. For great results, apply at night for smoother skin when you wake up.

A TASTE OF HONEY

Honey is well known for its antibacterial properties and ability to heal wounds, as well as its skin moisturizing and nourishing benefits. A natural humectant, it draws water to the skin. Mixed with olive oil and brown sugar it makes an effective skin exfoliant. It can also be used as a face mask, or with olive oil as a hair mask.

MAKE YOUR OWN TALC

Since talcum powder has been linked to an increased risk of ovarian cancer , it's better to make your own, natural version. A simple body powder can be made by mixing one cup of cornflour (cornstarch) with 10 to 30 drops of essential oil of your choice such as lavender or ylang ylang.

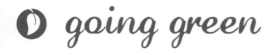 *going green*

HAVE A CLEAR OUT

Take a look at your bathroom cabinet and clear out everything but the essentials. If you've got more than one of any particular cosmetic product, pass it on, get rid of it and try not to buy duplicate products in the future.

CUT DOWN ON THE CREAMS

Why buy 20 different products when a few would do the job just as well? Start by asking yourself whether you really do need a separate hand, eye cream and moisturizer. Decide on a few key products such as a moisturizer, a sunscreen and a natural cleanser and stick to these.

BE ANIMAL-FRIENDLY

Vegetarians and vegans should be aware that make-up often contains a number of different animal ingredients. These include stearic acid and glycerin, sorbitan or octyl stearate, cochineal/carmine and silk. Vegans should also look out for beeswax, honey and lanolin. Animal-friendly brands include Dr Hauschka and The Body Shop.

SOLAR SHAVING

Invest in a solar-powered shaver for the ultimate in green shaving. The Sol-Shaver, a solar-powered shaver, has an integrated solar panel and needs to be left out in the sun to charge first. Ideal for travel and camping trips as well as everyday, energy-free shaving, you can charge it on a windowsill, outside in the sun – or even on the dashboard of your car.

MISS A WASH (OR TWO)

If you usually wash your hair every day, try leaving it for two or three days instead. Over-washing hair with chemical-based shampoos and conditioners can strip it of its natural oils. Once you have got used to the new regime you will probably find that your hair looks better and can be left for even longer between washes.

BARE-FACED CHEEK

Try going make-up free for one or two days a week to give your skin a chance to recover and breathe, especially if you are a regular wearer of pore-blocking cosmetics like foundation. Being bare-faced will also help reduce your exposure to chemicals.

CHOOSE LESS VIVID COLOURS FOR YOUR MAKE-UP

They are pretty but at what cost? A general rule of thumb when it comes to cosmetics is that the brighter the colour of a particular cosmetic, the more toxic it is likely to be. By choosing more neutral shades you will be helping to reduce demand for the most environmentally unfriendly pigments.

MAKE-UP WITH MINERALS

Mineral make-up, based on titanium and zinc oxide, has virtually no allergy risk, acts as an anti-inflammatory for sensitive skin, doesn't contain any fillers and contains natural sunscreens. It is particularly good for people with sensitive skin or those suffering from acne, rosacea or post-surgery. Good brands are Lily Lolo, Jane Iredale and Purity Cosmetics.

SUPPORT COMPACT FOR SAFE COSMETICS

Choose cosmetics brands where the manufacturers have signed up to the Compact for Safe Cosmetics campaign, which is run by the US-based Environmental Working Group. Each company pledges not to use chemicals that may cause cancer or birth defects in their products and to replace any hazardous materials with safer alternatives. For more information on the brands who partake in the campaign, visit www.safecosmetics.org/companies.

STAY AT HOME

Instead of travelling to the salon to get your legs waxed, use one of the natural home-waxing kits available. Look for one that doesn't require heating – therefore no extra energy – and that is made of natural ingredients. Nad's (www.nads.com) makes a version with molasses, honey and lemon.

CHOOSE NATURAL DEODORANTS

Deodorants often contain antibacterial ingredients and fragrance to minimize the odour-producing bacteria created by sweat. However, these ingredients often include triclosan, a known irritant, and parabens. Instead, choose natural deodorants containing essential oils for fragrance, with natural antibacterial properties.

NATURALLY ROUGH

Use an organic cotton muslin face cloth as part of your skincare regime. As well as having less environmental impact than conventional cotton, organic muslins will also be better for your skin. They act as a very gentle natural exfoliant to remove dead skin cells without causing irritation.

BUY VEGETABLE OIL SOAPS

Look for vegetable soaps made using the traditional cold-processing method which involves low energy, hand-crafted techniques. These soaps tend to be more suitable for people with sensitive skins and also allergy sufferers as they contain no additives. Caurnie soaps from Scotland also use a double saponification process to produce extra-gentle cleaning products.

PETROCHEMICAL-FREE CANDLES

Vegetable-based or beeswax candles are better for the environment and better for your health. When lit, normal paraffin candles emit trace amounts of toxins including formaldehyde and petroleum soot. Choose vegetable-based candles such as soy candles perfumed with pure essential oils for a greener alternative.

CHOOSE LOCAL AND HANDMADE

An increasing number of small manufacturers making handmade beauty care products using natural and organic ingredients. The production methods are usually small scale so have minimal environmental impact, and local production also cuts down on carbon emissions caused by transportation.

HAVE A SHOWER RATHER THAN A BATH

A bath uses around 170 litres (45 gallons) of water compared with 80 litres (21 gallons) for a five-minute shower. Therefore, switching from your daily bath to a shower can save over 32,000 litres (8,000 gallons) of water a year. Also a shower uses only 40% of the hot water necessary for a bath.

WISE UP

Most people think that ingredients in personal care and cosmetic products are safety tested before they are sold but there is no such requirement under federal law in the US. Ingredients including mercury, lead and even placenta have found their way into cosmetics.

LOOK OUT FOR ORGANIC

The global market for organic cosmetics is growing. However, be cautious: manufacturers are not legally required to obtain organic certification to make organic claims. Make sure the products you buy carry the logos of either the Soil Association, Ecocert or USDA Organic (United States Department of Agriculture). These products contain ingredients that are assessed to be safe to human health and guarantee that their manufacture and use causes minimum environmental impact.

NOT JUST SKIN DEEP

The outer layer of our skin can be penetrated quite well by some oils, which are often used in products to carry the active ingredients into the deeper layers of the skin. Therefore, it makes sense to give more consideration to the products that you apply and leave on the skin.

BEWARE THE COCKTAIL EFFECT

Research has found that the use of chemicals in cosmetics cannot be viewed in isolation. Because similar chemicals are found in a wide range of everyday items, as well as cosmetics, a cocktail effect is developing. The Women's Environmental Network says these chemicals are building up in, and damaging, the environment.

HEMP FOR BEAUTY

Hemp oil is an ideal ingredient for skin products because it is so rich in a unique balance of omega 3 and 6 oils. It is absorbed directly into the skin, nourishing and moisturizing it. Because it is a low-maintenance crop it doesn't require pesticides or fertilizers making it an ideal crop for sustainable farming.

SHOW YOUR SENSITIVE SIDE

Around 40% of the British population is now affected by allergies and, according to Allergy UK, over-exposure to chemicals can trigger a sensitivity that may lead to an allergy such as asthma, eczema or hay fever. Choosing natural products will reduce your exposure to chemicals.

BEAUTY MINEFIELD

Titanium oxide, which is a common ingredient in many sunscreens, and talc have been linked to environmental damage during the mining process and manufacture. Avoid talc when possible because it has also been associated with health problems such as ovarian cancer.

CHOOSE NATURAL TO AVOID HARMFUL TOXINS

We absorb around 60% of what we put on our skin and the average woman comes into contact with as many as 175 different chemicals from the beauty products she uses every day. Choose natural products without synthetic or manmade ingredients to avoid the toxins.

USE PERFUME SPARINGLY

To cut back on chemicals, cut back on perfume. If you can't live without your favourite scent, try to reduce the number of times you apply it. Instead of spraying it on day and night, keep it for special occasions and nights out. There are a growing number of natural and organic perfumes on the market so look out for these.

CHOOSE SELF-TAN NOT SUNTAN

The sun's rays are one of the main reasons for premature ageing and they also increase the risk of developing skin cancer. The same is true for sunbeds. Research has found that people using sunbeds in their teens and twenties have a 75% increased risk of developing skin cancer. Manufacturers Lavera and Green People both do a natural self-tanning lotion.

CHOOSE ESSENTIAL OILS, NOT SYNTHETIC FRAGRANCES

Manufacturers of synthetic fragrance oils do not have to disclose the ingredients used in their making, so you really have no idea what they contain although they are subject to safety guidelines. They are cheaper than essential oils, though, so are often used in beauty and bodycare products.

DON'T MIX IT UP

Avoid combining different products together as this may encourage nitrosamines to form. Nitrosamines are contaminants accidentally formed in cosmetics, either during manufacture, or storage if certain ingredients are combined. There is no research to prove that they can cause cancer in humans but evidence exists that they are carcinogenic in animals.

STRENGTHEN NAILS NATURALLY

Conventional nail-strengthening products often contain formaldehyde, which many people are allergic to and which is also a known carcinogen. Strengthen nails naturally by taking supplements with essential fatty acids and biotin (one of the B vitamins), and by eating enough protein (your nails are made of the natural protein keratin). Keep your nails from drying out and splitting by moisturizing daily.

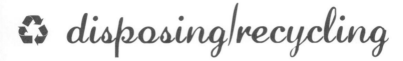

disposing/recycling

BUY PRODUCTS WITH RECYCLED PACKAGING
Packaging is one of the things used to sell cosmetics and beauty products, but it is unnecessary and adds to the growing global waste problem. Look for products that use recycled cardboard packaging such as those made by Living Nature and Lavera.

DISPOSE OF COTTON BUDS WISELY
Cotton buds (swabs) are one of the worst polluters of our seas, mainly because they are non-biodegradable, and yet lots of people flush them down the toilet rather than throwing them out as waste. Research by the Marine Conservation Society in the UK found that cotton buds are the second most-common polluter of beaches and seas.

USE REUSABLE PROTECTION
Well-designed reusable sanitary protection is now available, which helps reduce waste and cuts down on the environmental impact of sanpro production (many tampons also contain parabens, the oestrogen imitator that doesn't break down naturally). Organic feminine hygiene products can also reduce the health risks associated with conventional products.

USE RECYCLED FACIAL TISSUES
Around 3.2% of the world's commercial timber production goes into the manufacture of tissue products and Greenpeace estimates that an area of ancient forest the size of a football pitch disappears every two seconds in order to feed the demand for paper production. Buying recycled products helps to reduce illegal logging.

BUY IN BULK

It may not be the most glamorous option but try to buy products in the largest size available in order to cut back on packaging. You can then decant into a more convenient, smaller container at home. However, remember to check the shelf-life: you don't want to be left with products past the "best before" date.

TRAVEL LIGHT

Don't buy travel-sized versions of bodycare products when you are going on holiday. These containers are generally thrown away after use and end up on landfill. Instead, use your own small containers to decant your shampoo and shower gel, which can be rinsed out and re-used on your next trip.

RECYCLED COSMETIC BAGS

What better way to carry your cosmetics when travelling than in a recycled bag? A range of cosmetic and toiletry bags by Doy Bags are made from recycled juice packs by a women's cooperative in the Philippines. They can be bought from their website (www.doybags.com) and are shipped worldwide.

DITCH YOUR DISPOSABLE RAZORS

Men and women should avoid using disposable razors that are simply destined for the garbage bin. There's no need to purchase a product that has to be thrown away after a couple of uses – the emissions caused by their production and the waste created is completely avoidable. Invest in a decent razor and simply replace the blades when necessary.

BUY GLASS BOTTLES NOT PLASTIC

Packaging will contribute a great deal to the environmental impact
of all beauty and bodycare products. Therefore, where possible buy
products packaged in glass bottles rather than plastic as these are
easier to recycle. Good examples of this include deodorants from
Pitrok and Urtekram.

CHOOSE ORIGAMI-STYLE PAPER PACKAGING

A huge amount of the cost of a finished beauty product actually
goes on the packaging but some companies are changing their ways.
Pangea Organics' soap packaging is made from 100% post-consumer
newspaper. It is moulded using origami techniques so it doesn't
require glue and is infused with organic seeds.

REPLACE YOUR HEAD

Reduce plastic waste and landfill impact by using a toothbrush with
a replaceable head. Monte Blanco and Smile Brite brands do ranges
of replaceable head toothbrushes in various firmnesses for adults and
children that are no more expensive than standard brushes and work
out cheaper in the long run.

DON'T HAVE A SHOWER
JUST TO WASH YOUR HAIR

Water is a precious resource and one way to save a considerable
amount of it is not to have a bath or shower simply to wash your hair.
Use a hand-held shower attachment instead and turn the water off
while you apply the shampoo and conditioner.

DON'T BUY INTO PACKAGING

Research has revealed that as much as 50% of the cost of a bottle of
perfume can be accounted for by packaging and advertising. Some
companies offer a refill service where you can take in old bottles and
get them refilled, cutting back on waste and packaging.

USE A NATURAL SPONGE

Sea sponges are a non-endangered species and make a much greener alternative to synthetic sponges. Natural sea sponges also absorb a greater amount of water and clean more easily than synthetic varieties, resisting bacteria, mould and mildew. They are also longer lasting and more durable than manmade versions.

CHOOSE WOODEN BRUSHES

Avoid plastic brushes and choose wooden body brushes with natural-fibre bristles to clean nails and backs instead. Make sure that the wood comes from a sustainable source, and ideally is Forest Stewardship Council (FSC) certified. This also applies for toilet brushes.

RECYCLE OLD TOOTHBRUSHES

When you've finished with your toothbrush, give it a new lease of life. Toothbrushes make great scrubbing brushes for hard-to-reach corners and holes in and around the bathroom. They also make useful nailbrush substitutes.

CHOOSE YOUR TOOTHPASTE CAREFULLY

Toothpaste is one of the worst culprits when it comes to excessive packaging, with most relying on plastic tubes surrounded by cardboard containers. Look out for brands that use tubes made from biodegradable cellulose, such as Kingfisher, which has a range of natural toothpastes containing ingredients such as lemon, fennel and peppermint.

UNPLUG THE STRAIGHTENERS

Repeated use of hair straighteners can actually damage your hair, especially if it is fine. From an environmental perspective there is also the consideration of the energy used in their manufacture and during their use. Try to eliminate or reduce your reliance on hair straighteners, tongs, blow-dryers and other electric devices to reduce your carbon footprint and save the health of your hair.

shopping green

LOOK AT THE LABEL
Many of us are used to scanning food labels to check out salt and fat content and it is worth doing the same with cosmetics and beauty products. Lack of regulation means that literally hundreds of chemicals can be included in just one ingredient name – such as "fragrance".

BUY ORGANIC COTTON WOOL
Cotton production has a huge environmental impact due to the amount of chemicals used. A recent report found that cotton is responsible for the release of 15% of global insecticides, more than any other single crop. Buy certified organic cotton balls instead.

ORGANIC AWARENESS
A product carrying the Soil Association logo in the UK and the USDA Organic seal in the US must contain a minimum of 95% organic ingredients. However, a product that is labelled as "made with organic ingredients" must contain a minimum of 70% organic ingredients.

KNOWING IT'S NATURAL
One way to be sure that a European product is as natural as it claims to be is if it has been certified by the BDIH in Germany. This means the ingredients have to be from a plant or mineral source; most petroleum-based and synthetic ingredients are not permitted, and neither are GM ingredients.

GET ORGANICALLY LIPPY
The first certified organic lipstick in the UK was launched by Green People in 2006, following organic lipsticks by Nvey Eco and Hemp Organics in the US and Australia. Organic lippy is made using plant-based oils such as coconut and jojoba rather than petroleum-based ingredients. Green People's version contains fairly traded cupuaçu butter from the Brazilian Amazonian basin. See www.greenpeople. co.uk and www.econveybeauty.com for product information.

CHOOSE NATURAL NAIL POLISH

Conventional nail varnishes and removers are essentially cocktails of toxic chemicals, such as toluene and colour lakes (colour bases that don't break down in nature), acetone, formaldehyde and phthalates. Look for the BDIH label instead: this is a respected German association for certified natural cosmetics that guarantees a product based on plant oils and herbal and floral extracts from managed cultivation. The products it endorses do not include any organic-synthetic dyes, synthetic fragrances or mineral oil derivatives. Sante Natural Nail Polishes are certified by the BDIH.

KEEP AN EYE ON INGREDIENTS

Many mainstream eyeshadows contain coal tar, albeit in tiny amounts. Lipstick is another product that sometimes holds high levels of artificial colourings made from coal-tar derivatives. Coal tar has been linked to cancer and has been found to cause allergic reactions in some people.

CHOOSE A BIODEGRADABLE "BLOCK" SUNSCREEN

Sunscreens reduce the risk of skin cancer but they don't protect you from the sun's rays. Many contain chemicals that are not biodegradable but can wash off into the water supply, too. Most sunscreens offer a combination of both chemical and physical-barrier ingredients to protect you from the sun. Zinc oxide is the best physical-barrier screen as it has no harmful side-effects, no extra ingredients and is a mineral, so it is not absorbed into the bloodstream. Traditionally available in the thick white formula, there are now transparent versions.

GOOD ENOUGH TO EAT

A current trend in the beauty world is for making cosmetics using food-grade ingredients such as fruit, oats and vegetables that are designed to nourish your skin from the outside in. British cosmetic company NOe (Natural Organic edible) and US company Befine Food Skincare are good examples of this trend. Their products are natural and preservative-free.

AVOID PUMP-ACTION DISPENSERS

When buying toothpaste avoid the pump-action dispensers. These are really unnecessary and use even more plastic than regular tubes. They cannot be recycled easily and therefore end up on landfill sites where they won't decompose.

STICK TO THE SHELF-LIFE

Bear in mind that natural products won't contain the same levels of chemical preservatives as other brands, so their shelf life will be shorter. Always use products before their "best before" date and dispose of any after this time.

COMMON SCENTS

Look out for the word "fragrance" on ingredients lists. Current legislation doesn't restrict the quantities or combinations of fragrance chemicals that can be used in everyday cosmetics. This means that it's not unusual for some products to contain as much as between 50 and 100 fragrances.

AVOID MUSK FOR DEERS' SAKE

Many upmarket perfumes contain substances such as musk and civet. Musk comes from the gland of a male musk deer which has been hunted to near extinction. Civet is a secretion from civet cats and there are reports that they are tormented to increase the secretions they produce. Avoid fragrances containing these ingredients.

AVOID ARTIFICIAL COLOURS IN YOUR TOOTHPASTE

Look out for natural, SLS (sodium lauryl sulfate)-free toothpaste without added colours. There's no need for multicoloured stripes when you're brushing your teeth. Look for brands using natural ingredients such as fennel and peppermint, which have natural breath-freshening and antiseptic properties.

CHOOSE TO BE FRAGRANCE- FREE

Manufacturers are not legally required to list any of the potentially hundreds of chemicals in a single product's fragrance mixture. Fragrances can contain neurotoxins and are known allergens. Avoid them by choosing products fragranced only with pure essential oils.

ETHICAL BEAUTY

Manufacturers, by law, have to test their products and it is up to them how they do it, so use your purchasing power to send a message to cosmetics companies that testing on animals is unacceptable. The European Union has passed a ban on animal testing in cosmetics, starting in 2009 with a complete ban in 2013.

SAY NO TO TANNING PILLS

Tanning pills usually contain the pigment canthaxanthin, which is highly dangerous. Although approved for use in food in minimal amounts, in tanning pills it is ingested in high doses and works by changing not only the skin to an orange-brown colour, but also the internal organs. Canthaxanthin has been linked to hepatitis and canthaxanthin retinopathy (yellow deposits in the retina of the eye).

KNOW YOUR FOAMING AGENTS

Choose products containing plant-based foaming agents such as coconut oil and decyl glucoside, which is extracted from corn. These are preferable to sodium laurel sulphate (SLS), commonly used in bodycare products.

BE CAREFUL WHAT YOU WASH DOWN YOUR SINK

Triclosan, a common ingredient in toothpaste, deodorant and soap, is known to be environmentally harmful. It can be converted to cancer-causing dioxin when exposed to sunlight in water and has been classified as toxic to aquatic organisms and the aquatic environment.

CHOOSE PRODUCTS WITH FEWER INGREDIENTS

The more natural a product, the fewer ingredients it is likely to have. A good clue that a product is full of chemicals is the length of the ingredients list, so if in doubt avoid it. The more ingredients it contains, the more likely it is that you may react badly to one of them.

USE ESSENTIAL OILS

Choose products containing organic essential oils as many of them have the added benefit of acting as natural preservatives. Make sure you store them away from sunlight, preferably in dark glass bottles, and that way they will last longer.

PACK IN THE PETROLEUM PRODUCTS

Petroleum-based ingredients such as petrolatum, which is also known as baby oil, strips the natural oils from the skin, causing chapping and dryness, and even premature ageing. The manufacture of petroleum-based ingredients also has a major impact on the environment.

BUY FAIRTRADE COTTON WOOL

Make sure that your cotton wool isn't being produced at the expense of the workers creating it by buying Fairtrade-certified cotton wool and cotton buds (swabs). Look for the International Fairtrade Association FTO mark on products (see www.ifat.org). In the UK fairtrade products must be registered by the Fairtrade Foundation and carry the fairtrade mark (see www.fairtrade.org.uk).

HIGH IN HERBS

Herbs such as aloe vera and lavender have been traditionally used for their cleansing, moisturizing and soothing qualities. Products high in herbal content rather than synthetics are not only natural but also very effective. Look for organic or wild-crafted herbal products to ensure the environment is also being protected.

WHAT IS A NATURAL INGREDIENT?

A natural substance is any plant or animal extract, or any rock or mineral obtained from the earth. It is possible to make exact copies of natural substances using raw materials from coal tar and petroleum and many manufacturers choose to synthesize ingredients rather than to extract them from natural sources.

Mind & Body

FROM TIPS ON BOOSTING YOUR FITNESS and planning some "you" time to guidance on alternative therapies and coping with stress, this chapter is crammed full of expert advice on your overall wellbeing. With easy-to-follow solutions for sleep problems, relationship ruts, and nagging aches and pains, the following mind and body secrets will help you get your health and happiness back in balance.

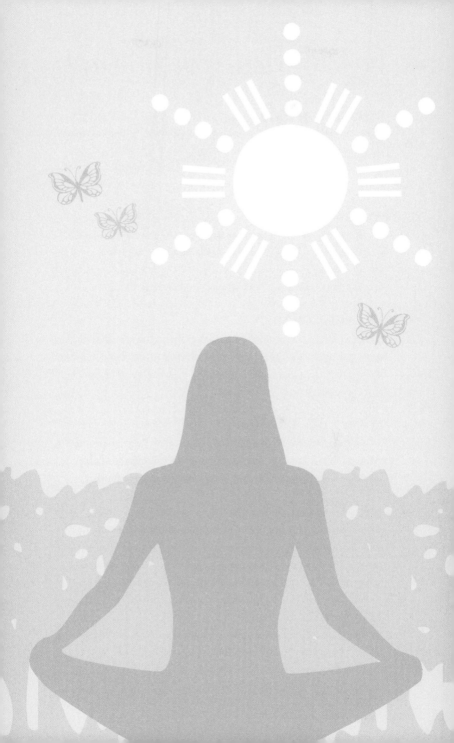

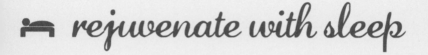# rejuvenate with sleep

THE HOURS
Sleep between the hours of 10pm and 6am if you can. The first four hours are when physical regeneration takes place. The second four bring mental and emotional recharging, so you wake up looking and feeling better.

AVOID STIMULANTS
Lack of sleep can have a negative impact on your body, mind and looks, leading to puffy, tired eyes and dull-looking skin. Avoid stimulants like alcohol, nicotine and caffeine late at night, as these all effect the nervous system and disrupt sleep patterns.

GET INTO A ROUTINE
A regular bedtime schedule will help your body to expect sleep at the same time each day. Spend quiet time relaxing in a warm bath infused with a few drops of essential lavender oil to soothe the mind and body and encourage regenerative sleep.

SLEEP LIKE AN ITALIAN
Starchy carbohydrates are vital for a healthy body, and an evening meal that has some carbohydrate content can help raise levels of seratonin – a brain chemical that helps control sleep patterns.

REGENERATION FUNDS
Scientists know that relaxation is a restorative time for the body, when the body repairs and regenerates itself. It is during its relaxed state that the brain produces "feel-good molecules", immunity is boosted and the body repairs and forms new tissue.

NOISE POLLUTION
One of the biggest distractions to getting a good night's sleep is noise. Try to cut out night-time noise when you go to bed, even if it means wearing ear plugs. Sleep is a regenerative time, but you need some uninterrupted hours for your body to restore itself.

DRINK UP AT BEDTIME

A hot milky drink at bedtime is good because it contains the amino acid L-tryptophan, a precursor of the sleep inducing hormones melatonin and serotonin.

DOWNLOAD FIRST

If you have difficulty nodding off because the worries of the day are still rushing around in your head, get out of bed and write a list of everything that's bothering you, and a to-do list if necessary. Once you have unloaded your brain, you should be able to sink into a regenerative sleep.

SIMULATE MELATONIN

Ageing can blur your waking and sleeping patterns, but numerous researchers have found that the hormone melatonin can enhance longevity, promote deep and restful sleep, slow cell damage and ageing, as well as support the immune system and improve energy levels. Enhance your natural levels of melatonin by always going to sleep in the dark.

NOD OFF NATURALLY

The herb valerian has been used in traditional sleep remedies for hundreds of years. It is thought to relieve anxiety and to aid the induction of sleep in a natural and non-addictive way.

FIND THE RIGHT POSITION

Learn to sleep on your back – it's the best position for relaxing and it allows all your internal organs to rest properly.

REPAIR THE BRAIN

According to research by Princeton University for the World Health Organization, missing out on sleep may cause the brain to stop producing new cells and can negatively affect the part of the brain called the hippocampus, which is responsible for forming memories. Middle-aged people should get seven hours a night – you know you are getting enough when you wake spontaneously without an alarm clock.

SWEET FRESH SLEEP

Good sleep comes in a room that has a window ajar. Unexpected odours disrupt sleep patterns, increasing the heart rate and quickening brain waves. Sprinkle some heliotropine, a vanilla-almond fragrance, on your pillow to help promote a good night's sleep.

PILLOW PRESSURE

Reduce stress and tension by resting on a thermal neck pillow that can be heated up in the microwave. The heat generated by the pillow penetrates into the tense neck muscles, soothing away aches and pains and relieving headaches and those oh-so ageing frowns.

COPY THE CONTINENTALS

The Mediterranean habit of a siesta has enormous health benefits as we get older. A "disco nap" between the hours of 3pm and 5pm, where you take off your clothes and get properly into bed, will leave you with more energy, alertness and enthusiasm for the evening ahead.

LULL WITH LAVENDER

Place a small lavender-filled pillow in your bed to promote a restful night's sleep. The herb is thought to reduce levels of anxiety and promote general feelings of wellbeing.

 relaxing & de-stressing

CD MEANS CALM DOWN

To reduce stress or that panicky feeling of having far too much to do, buy a hypnotherapy CD. Lie down and listen to a calming voice, letting all your worries drift away and reducing the chaos in your mind – your face will relax too!

GET HELP

Seek professional help if you feel consumed by anger, jealousy or guilt. These emotions are "poisonous" to a healthy mind and body, and could eventually lead to stress-related illnesses.

GOAL-ORIENTATED VISUALIZATION

Sit quietly for 5 minutes a day in a calm meditative state where you visualize yourself in any situation of warmth and happiness to get rid of urban stress, tension and anxiety – all of which cause headaches and frown lines.

ACCENTUATE THE POSITIVE

Cognitive behavioural therapy (CBT) believes that negative attitudes and beliefs are unhealthy modes of thinking that have been learned over a long time. It challenges this way of thinking and encourages you to take a more positive and assertive view.

BAN NEGATIVE WORDS

Words like "can't", "won't" and "shouldn't" all have negative connotations that make you think in a pessimistic way. Take a more positve approach – studies have shown that optimists are healthier people who have higher levels of antibodies and greater energy.

GO DEEPER WITHIN

Shut off from the material world and practice meditation. Sitting cross-legged for just 10 minutes a day, listening to your own breath, each inhale and exhale, and letting go of your emotional baggage will calm a stressed mind and body and give you better perspective.

AN END TO CONFLICT

Arguments and hostility lead to an endless release of the stress hormone cortisol. The hormone raises blood sugar, and high levels of excess cortisol lead to excess fat being deposited on the body, particularly around the tummy area. No one can avoid conflict completely, but investigate some cognitive behavioural techniques to reduce the negative feelings conflict brings.

MAKE TIME FOR YOU

Spending time quietly alone, where you can empty your mind of all your thoughts, learn to focus and begin to feel a calm awareness of the world around you, will provide physical and mental health benefits, if you do it regularly.

CHANTING FOR THE INNER YOU

Meditative chanting can diminish all negative feelings such as anger, envy, boredom and greed. The process encourages a kind of inner happiness brought about by the transcendental sound vibrations of chanting.

GET A FURRY FRIEND

As stress-busters go, this is one of the nicest ways to lift your mood and relieve stress, as long as you're not allergic to dogs! Bad moods disappear with a furry puppy on your lap – they provide companionship and unconditional love, and they encourage you to get outdoors.

TAKE SOME TIME OUT

Book a week away from it all at a country retreat, spa or religious centre, where you can take advantage of complementary therapies and treatments. You will experience the benefits of relaxation, develop inner strength and refresh your mind and body away from daily stresses.

confidence tricks

GET IN TOUCH WITH YOURSELF

Become more self aware and get in touch with your inner feelings so that you can identify different emotions. An easy visualization technique is to blank the mind and think only of blue sky, and a white sandy beach. Imagine you are in that sunny situation and how it feels.

ISOLATE YOUR MUSCLES

Get into the habit of using relaxation techniques such as progressive muscle relaxation, where you tense, hold for 10 seconds then release each muscle group one by one. Used regularly it can improve your immune system and coping skills, as well as significantly reducing the likelihood of a heart attack.

TOO MUCH INFORMATION

Most of us are overstimulated. Resolve to not watch TV or buy any newspapers for a week. Turn off your mobile for at least a few hours every day and limit home time on email to the weekends.

RESOLVE TO RELAX

Clean your body and your mind, and let yourself have a few minutes of uninterrupted time in a relaxing bath. Add skin-softening milk, and let yourself drift off, letting the problems of the day float away with the bubbles.

FORM A LASTING IMPRESSION

Remember that after the first ten seconds, most people won't judge you on the way you look. If your inner beauty shines through you will make a good impression and people will respond positively to you.

MAKE LIKE A MOVIE STAR

Like anything else, beauty needs to be "sold". Try deliberately looking and acting more confident. If you add extra zing to the way you come across, people will respond to you more positively – and that in turn will make you feel even better about yourself.

RECRUIT SOME BOOSTERS

Instead of filling your bathroom with expensive beauty treatments, surround yourself with some different confidence boosters – your friends. If you spend time with people who tell you how beautiful you are, you will soon feel – and see – the positive effects.

FAKE IT

Just as applying your favourite lipstick can make a difference to your mood, the first step to feeling better about yourself is often to start acting confidently, even if you're feeling down. Act like you feel beautiful and people will respond to that self-confidence.

IGNORE THE COMPETITION

Nothing ruins a beautiful face like a frown, so don't make comparisons that will only make you miserable. In particular, don't compare yourself with the celebrities you see in the magazines – their pics are airbrushed so what you see is not real!

MAKE A HEALTHY CHOICE

The health benefits of having a nutritious salad and a glass of water for lunch are not immediately apparent, but if you're feeling low the confidence-boosting effects can be beneficial. Feeling like you've given your body a healthy treat makes you feel instantly better about yourself, which is a great beauty pick-me-up.

SEIZE THE DAY

Make an effort to look good every day and you'll instantly feel more attractive. Give yourself enough time to blow-dry your hair, apply a touch of make-up and pick out your most stylish and brightly coloured clothes.

TAKE UP SPACE

Don't spend money on your make-up and clothes only to disappear into a corner at social functions. Allow yourself to take centre stage with broad gestures and a clear, definite voice tone.

FIVE-SECOND FIX

If you ever find yourself feeling bad about the way you look, use this quick strategy: remember a time when you felt really confident in your appearance, then take a deep breath and as you let it out, allow yourself to feel good.

STAND TALL

A confident posture costs nothing and is better than an expensive new outfit. Hold your head high and keep your shoulders back. Place your feet hip-width apart so that you're well balanced and maintain eye contact with the other person.

A SEXY SECRET

Underwear doesn't have to be seen by anyone else to be special. You can add a sexy swagger to your walk simply by wearing your favourite underwear under your work clothes.

GIVE TO RECEIVE

Remember, the best way to get that beauty-enhancing confidence boost you require is to compliment others. Make an effort to tell people you meet or work with how great they look, especially when they've made an effort or look unhappy. That way people will think to return the compliment when you need it the most.

ACCENTUATE THE POSITIVE

Too much make-up focuses on fixing the bits you don't like about your face. It's much more rewarding to find something you do like about your face – perhaps you have great bone structure or a rosebud mouth? Now concentrate on playing up these good bits.

TELL YOURSELF YOU'RE BEAUTIFUL

A self-compliment may sound cheesy, but there's no point spending lots of money on make-up if you don't believe you're worth it. The first step to being beautiful is feeling good about yourself, so get rid of the inner-critic and say something positive.

BOOST YOUR CONFIDENCE

Believing in your own good looks will make others believe in them, too. Presenting a positive mental attitude and self-assurance will help you exude attractiveness. If you don't always feel it, try pretending to be confident and good-looking – it can make a big difference to how others perceive you.

TAKE A BREAK FROM YOURSELF

Role-play doesn't have to be limited to the bedroom – or require an audience. You can get a real beauty boost just by pretending to be someone else for a day. There's no need to tell anyone – just do your make-up differently, change your style of dress, maybe even wear a wig.

CHANGE IT UP

If you always play safe and stick to the same make-up routine, the positive effects will start to wear off after a while. There's no need to buy new make-up; just use what you've got a little differently – wear your eyeliner a little thicker or gloss your lips after applying lipstick.

GO NATURAL

Have the confidence to leave the house without any make-up on. It will reduce your dependence on too many products and save you money. Start with a trip to the supermarket.

BREATHE YOURSELF BEAUTIFUL

Breathing properly is key to beautiful skin, hair and nails because it encourages higher levels of oxygen into your system. To ensure you're breathing deeply, place your hands on your belly and feel it expand as you take an in-breath, and deflate as you breathe out naturally.
To start each day relaxed and calm, take a few minutes each morning to close your eyes and concentrate on your breathing.

think yourself younger

PRACTISE MEMORY GAMES

Keep the brain healthy by exercising your failing memory. Directly after a social occasion, re-live the event in your head – the plot of the movie or play, the costumes or set. Or if you were at a party, try to recall individual details about the people you met. Use visual clues to help you remember – the stranger and more unusual, the more likely it is you will be able to recall the associated information later on.

STOP BRAIN-CELL DECLINE

After the age of 35, brain cells die off at a rate of 100,000 per day and are not replaced. Meditation can reduce this decaying process as it changes the vibratory make-up of the mind.

ROAR LIKE A LION

Use the yoga position called the Lion to keep your face and neck vibrant and toned. Take a deep breath and, as you breathe out, open your mouth as wide as possible and stick out your tongue. Move your eyes (but not your head) to look at the ceiling, without straining them, and hold for a count of eight.

BE A MULTITASKER

According to a study at Trinity College, Dublin, juggling many tasks at once helps to keep your mind young and active. As we age we challenge ourselves mentally less and less, and the effort involved in keeping several things to the forefront of your mind at once exercises the brain.

USE IT OR LOSE IT

Keep challenging yourself mentally to learn a new skill, take up a new hobby or read more books. Research has shown that brain cells need to be exercised in the same way that the physical body does to keep fit and healthy.

BINGO BOOSTS BRAIN CELLS

Keeping the brain mentally active is thought to help maintain mental alertness. Bingo players have been found to be faster and more accurate in tests than non-bingo players, and mental agility is believed to stave off depression and degenerative brain disease.

KEEP NOTE OF YOUR FIVE SENSES

Practice a daily mental workout to avoid sluggish thinking and memory loss; mental decline with old age is not inevitable if the brain remains busy. Make-up your own exercises to strengthen all five senses – sight, sound, smell, taste and touch – and keep a record to note down week-by-week enhancements of each.

CHEW GUM FOR MEMORY

Studies show that chewing gum can improve long-term and working memory. The chewing action increases heart rate, improving the delivery of oxygen and nutrients to the brain, and triggers the release of insulin, which may stimulate memory.

FOCUS YOUR MIND ON A HOBBY

Our brains naturally start slowing down at the age of 30. However, studies show that people of any age can train their brains to be faster and, in effect, younger. Experts say that any hobby that closely engages your focus and is strongly rewarding will kick your brain into learning mode and notch it up.

STAY CONNECTED

Make a concerted effort to keep up-to-date with technological advances. Get an iPod and download some current music tracks or podcasts, or log onto YouTube or MySpace. Don't try to compete with younger people – just keep abreast of trends and make sure you know what they're talking about.

CROSS WORDS

Research has shown that keeping the mind agile is just as important as keeping fit in the battle to stay young. A lazy brain needs exercising in the same way that the body does. Try to do a crossword puzzle or play a game of Sudoku every day to stimulate brain cells and keep them active and healthy. Other claimed benefits include the delay or prevention of Alzheimer's disease.

GET EDUCATED

Many of us who would like to learn a new language or master a musical instrument are put off by the fact that we will not be as "quick" as we were when we were kids. But research has proved that the greater our education – no matter when we achieved it – the more likely we are to live long and fulfilled lives.

HAVE AN ADVENTURE

Remember how the world seemed like such an exciting place and you couldn't wait to explore it? There's no need to lose that feeling just because you're a little bit older. Book an adventure holiday, such as a trek in another country, or go somewhere you've never been before. Eat the local food and immerse yourself in the culture – you will go a long way towards stimulating your mind and helping yourself to feel active and youthful.

LEARN TO LOVE WHAT YOU HATE

Taking up a task or skill you've never particularly enjoyed is a good way to address lazy thought patterns. For example, if you've never enjoyed history, try memorizing some facts, or if you have a block about maths, exercise accounting skills. Going against type will invigorate the mind and prevent predictable ways of thinking.

SET GOALS

If you want to make changes in your life it helps to set achievable goals. There are no quick fixes to roll back the ravages of time, but changing bad habits and looking at lifestyle changes will give you a positive outlook for the future.

A DIFFERENT PATH

Changing your daily habits slightly will help you keep a fresh perspective. For example, vary the route you take to walk to work, and take some time to notice the different surroundings. If you drive a car, take a longer route occasionally, or if you always have lunch at a specific time, take it an hour later.

SPEAK IN TONGUES

Learning a second language forces your brain to switch tracks continuously, which is one of the most mentally demanding things you can do. It's particularly effective for honing the frontal lobes – the brain's mind manager – which generally shrink with age.

SCARE YOURSELF SILLY

Everyone slips into safe routines and situations. To keep young, you need to be aware that this may not help you grow and develop – which is important at any age. Try doing something that frightens you a little – it could be as challenging as parachuting or bungee jumping, or simply having a weekend away on your own.

COGNITIVE POWERS OF THE FUTURE

Ampakines, a class of drugs that enhance learning, memory and concentration, are being developed; they also aid Alzheimer's, Parkinson's and other age-related mental disabilities.

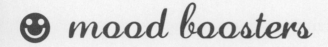 # mood boosters

PUT ON A HAPPY FACE
Nothing is more attractive than someone with a happy smile – it makes you look young, fun and carefree. Research has shown that people who practise fake smiling actually end up feeling happier as a result – just as those who practise frowning feel more depressed.

KEEP A SUNNY OUTLOOK
Don't let yourself become overanxious to the point that fears and worries dominate your whole life. A worried mind is not at peace and it will deplete energy levels, which you need to maintain youthfulness.

THINK HAPPY
Learn to be happy within yourself, and not to compare your life, looks or financial situation with others. No amount of surgery, needles or scalpels will change the way you feel inside. An optimistic nature, a network of supportive friends and some feeling of control over your life are some of the most important things for graceful, stress-free ageing.

IMPROVE MOOD WITH SELENIUM
When US Department of Agriculture (USDA) researchers fed young men a diet that contained 220 mcg of the mineral selenium per day (the average American diet has 40 to 60 mcg), the men reported feeling elated, clearheaded, confident and energetic.

GRUMPY OLD GALS
We all make excuses about why we eat the wrong foods, don't have enough time to exercise and drink too much alcohol. The truth is we do have the power to change the things we dislike about our lives. A commitment to making small changes can lead to a healthier and more fulfilling life.

FALL IN LOVE

Maybe easier to say than to do, but falling in love produces a surge of feel-good endorphins in the brain (dopamine, norepinephrine and phenylethylamine), which are responsible for uncontrollable feelings of euphoria. This huge chemical hit inside the brain gives you flushed cheeks and a racing heart, and will make you look and feel five years younger. If the real deal proves elusive, cultivate crushes and flirt – it will still trigger that rush of endorphins and you'll have lots of fun in the process!

GIVE BLOOD

Rolling up your sleeve and donating blood to help save someone else's life will remind you that there are others more needy than you. You will also benefit from having your blood pressure, pulse and haemoglobin levels checked.

BRAIN FOOD

People who eat breakfast are happier, and studies have proved that early morning food has beneficial effects on mental and physical functions. The body needs to refuel after sleep, and breakfast eaters have higher concentration levels in the morning.

BEAUTY FROM WITHIN

Comparing yourself to supermodels, movie stars or even the yummy mummy on the school run is not a good idea. Stop worrying what other people think of you. Real beauty is about confidence and not about achieving a certain size of figure or attaining wealth. Start feeling good about yourself and you will begin to radiate an inner beauty.

GOOD MORNING

Be happier by getting up earlier in the morning. Researchers from the University of California have found that early-morning light raised levels of luteinizing hormone (LH) by up to 70%. This hormone can help to build muscle, cut fat and raise mood.

FOCUS ON THE POSITIVE

Emotion researchers have discovered that as people get older, they experience fewer negative emotions and report better control over their emotions – they also tend to enhance positive memories and diminish negative ones. Mirror this "positivity effect" by dismissing every negative thought that comes your way.

BE HAPPY-GO-LUCKY

People who maximize opportunities, are open to new experiences and act instinctively are more likely to create their own luck, increase their self-esteem and generate a positive energy.

THE KARMA OF KINDNESS

Being kind to others has positive health benefits both physically and mentally. A rush of euphoria, followed by a longer period of calm is known as the "helper's high" which can trigger feel good endorphins into the body and help ease depression.

YOUNG AT HEART

Make sure your social group of friends includes some who are much younger. Having young friends who have a less cynical and more optimistic approach to life will keep energy levels high, and make you feel and look younger.

GRAB A LITTLE LOVING

Feelings of love and trust between a couple and a healthy sex life have been scientifically proved to make you feel good all over. Good sex releases endorphins in the brain that create an overall level of contentment. It can also act as a natural tranquillizer that calms you down and promotes good sleep, as well as making you feel fit, healthy and younger. So what's stopping you!

WATCH A WEEPY

Research has shown that it's good to have a good cry now and again. Tears appear to reduce tension, remove toxins and increase the body's ability to heal itself. After an outburst of tears the body is flooded with oxygen, which triggers the release of feel-good hormones in the brain.

FIND SOMEONE TO CUDDLE

Research shows that cuddling decreases levels of stress hormones and boosts levels of serotonin in the brain. Regular cuddles can stimulate the production of feel-good endorphins and oxytocin, making you feel and look happier and younger.

BEAT THE BLUES

If you're prone to depression take preventative action with a course of the herbal remedy St John's Wort (hypericum). In clinical trials it has proved successful in helping to lift mild depression and calm anxiety. It's a good idea to consult a health professional first though.

HAVE A GOOD CHAT

Interacting with others can bring about a deep sense of relaxation and happiness for women. Recent studies have proven that the act of talking triggers a flood of chemicals – which (scientists say) gives women a rush similar to that felt by heroin addicts on a high!

HAVE A GIGGLE

Laughter may be the best medicine after all, as it has been shown to increase blood flow by more than 20% – similar to that of aerobic activity. So a good laugh at a comedy movie may help fight infections, ease pain and control diabetes. It has also been shown that people who laugh daily have stronger immune systems and live longer.

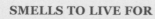

SMELLS TO LIVE FOR

Make yourself feel extra special by spritzing on a new scent or using a room spray or scented candles in the home. Fragrances can be very powerful memory triggers that can take you back to a special time and place where you can re-live happy memories. They are also relaxants.

NUTURE YOUR RELATIONSHIP

Studies have shown that people who are married or in a loving relationship reduce their risk of illness by 50%. Married couples live longer, are less stressed and are said to have fewer heart attacks than single people.

THE SOUND OF MUSIC

If you're feeling blue, turn on your favourite CD, and have your own private karaoke session! The physical act of loud singing, combined with the rhythmic breathing it entails, will make you feel much better about yourself.

DOWN AND DIRTY

Spend an afternoon potting and pruning to put yourself into a good mood and relieve tension. Reconnecting with the earth and nature has a calming effect on stress levels, and strenuous digging will give you a fabulous rosy glow.

SEIZE THE DAY

Make every day count, and at the end of it you will feel more content and peaceful within yourself. Wear new clothes, drink that bottle of champagne and don't save your special perfume for best.

DON'T WORRY, BE HAPPY

Stress and worry cause frowning, and over time the muscles in the face actually conform to that movement and stress wrinkles are formed. Be aware of your stress levels and try to vary your facial expressions during the day – laughter is both a good stress buster and a great way to avoid wrinkles.

SAY IT WITH FLOWERS

Research from Texas A&M University found that flowers and plants could help to raise spirits and improve levels of creativity and feelings of happiness. A few bunches of fragrant flowers can be enough to scent your home and lift your mood for days.

EAT A HAPPY MEAL

Food can directly affect the neurotransmitter chemicals in your brain responsible for maintaining an elevated mood. For the best mood boost, combine lean proteins with complex carbohydrates. Ease up on saturated fats and convenience foods.

BECAUSE YOU'RE WORTH IT

Because women are great providers, they often lose sight of their own needs. It's important to make time in the week to do something for yourself – stay in contact with friends, go and watch a movie, or take up a new hobby. Finding something that makes you happy will increase your confidence and general feelings of wellbeing.

SLOW DOWN

Living at breakneck speed and using stimulants like caffeine and alcohol to boost levels of adrenaline is very damaging to the body. It lowers immunity and weakens the digestive system, as well as triggering mood swings. Make time for yourself each day to contemplate life.

GET CREATIVE WITH SCENT

Sweet-smelling perfume is thought to help boost creativity and encourage problem solving. Dab your favourite scent on to your wrists and collarbones, but not behind your ears as the oily skin there interferes with the fragrance.

basic fitness principles

MAINTAINING GOOD HEALTH

It's a sad fact that with every decade that passes, metabolic rate drops and fat-burning muscles reduce. To maintain the same body weight and shape you will have to increase your exercise routine and eat slightly smaller portions. It's worth remembering that 0.5 kg (1 lb) of fat is the equivalent of 3,500 calories. So if you find it easy to put on weight, look seriously at your food and exercise regime.

TIGHTEN UP WITH KEGEL EXERCISES

After childbirth or the menopause you may find your pelvic floor muscles not quite up to the job, and experience an embarrassing little leakage when you cough, laugh or go jogging. You can tighten the muscles, either by sucking in, and tensing up as if you were trying to hold a stream of urine, or with a clever device called the Pelvic Toner.

EXERCISE FOR BRAIN HEALTH

Moderate exercise can help prevent slowing processes that come with age, as it enhances blood flow to the brain (which can reduce the risk of stroke), improves cognitive processing, and slows down the degeneration of the nervous system. Don't think of exercise as a short-term punishment that you have to "put up with", make it a part of your daily routine – and after a couple of weeks it will become second nature to you. Laying down a good habit when you are younger will help you continue throughout your senior years.

GO FOR THE BURN

For exercise to be beneficial you need to raise your heartbeat, which will improve circulation and metabolism. Sweating is also good as it encourages the production of sebum which acts as the skin's own natural moisturizer.

BUILD UP HIGH

Many useful hormones in the body that help maintain energy levels, metabolic rate, and control healthy body function can be boosted by moderate exercise. Exercise acts as a major stimulus for the natural secretion of human growth hormone (hGH) and some studies have found that increased hGH, testosterone and endorphins can increase longevity and help to reverse the ageing process.

LOSE A LITTLE FOR BIG BENEFITS

Whatever your weight, you only have to lose a little to see massive health benefits. Losing just 5–10% of your body weight will lower blood pressure, cut your risk of diabetes and heart disease, and lower your intake of bad cholesterol. And there is evidence that lower weight corresponds to greater longevity. Losing body fat and creating lean muscles will also give you an improved overall body shape, while extra muscle gives you better posture and much more energy.

LIVE LONG AND WELL

According to a recent study in the American Journal of Sports Medicine, the "greatest threat to health is not the ageing process itself but inactivity." Moderate physical exercise has been proven to delay the effects of ageing, even if you only start it later in life, and possibly increase longevity. The study clearly demonstrated that regular vigorous exercise of just 30 minutes a day is associated with increased life expectancy. Several other studies have shown that colon cancer is reduced 30% in individuals who exercise regularly.

⨍ aerobic exercise

HIT THE DANCE FLOOR
You're never too old to make a statement on the dance floor; it's good exercise to keep the body loose. Dancing will bring a youthful flush to the cheeks that is only achieved by running 3 miles or having great sex.

A QUICK STEP TO FITNESS
The simple act of walking will bring significant benefits to your heart and weight. A brisk walk that raises the metabolic rate and makes you a little short of breath will also bring a fresh, rosy glow to your cheeks. Buy a clip-on pedometer that can measure your body fat, and aim to walk 10,000 steps a day.

UGLY VEINS NEED A SHAKE UP
About 40% of women suffer from ugly varicose veins. Regular aerobic exercise several times a week will get the muscles working. It will also get the blood pumping through the tiny valves to make the condition much less noticeable.

FIGHT CELLULITE WITH FITNESS
Few female athletes have cellulite because exercise replaces body fat with muscle, and prevents fat cells from becoming blocked with toxins. Jogging, swimming, cycling and walking are all excellent ways to improve circulation and encourage the elimination of toxins.

SMASHING SQUASH
Bashing a tiny rubber ball around a court has to be one of the most energetic things you can do with a friend or on your own. The smashing action is a great stress buster, and a 30-minute game of squash will leave you with better aerobic fitness, as well as toning and strengthening all muscle groups.

BE AEROBIC FOR FULL-BODY HEALTH

Aerobic exercise provides an overwhelming number of benefits that help in keeping the body functioning as it did when you were younger, including: boosting circulation; keeping the heart, arteries and veins healthy; perking up the mood and enhancing brain function; helping you sleep; improving digestion and immunity; and enhancing your skin and general appearance.

STEADY SKIPPING

It's so easy even a child can do it, but skipping is a tough calorie-burning workout that is difficult to sustain for 10 minutes. Try to keep your knees bent at all times, barely lifting your feet off the ground, and flicking the rope over your head.

BREAK INTO A RUN

Walking is good for you but jogging is even better. If you've never jogged a step, then start with walking and jogging alternatively, five minutes each for 30 minutes total. Gradually increase the ratio of jogging to walking until it becomes the total exercise time.

GET ON YOUR BIKE

Despite what you may think, cyclists absorb lower levels of pollutants from traffic fumes than car drivers, and if you cycle regularly, research has shown you can expect to be as fit as an average person 10 years younger.

BOUNCE AWAY PAIN

Mini rebounders that fit inside your bedroom provide a great aerobic workout for all levels of fitness and ages, though older people will need to do gentler, less gymnastic moves. Rebounding protects joints from hard-impact exercise and offers relief from neck and back pains. It also strengthens leg muscles and increases oxygen availability throughout the body.

NO WATER NEEDED

The advantage of a rowing machine is that it offers an all-over workout with very little impact on joints. Vigorous rowing is one of the most effective calorie-burning exercises, but you can set your own pace, and it will tone up flabby arms and help give you a flatter stomach.

RELIEF FOR BACK PAIN

Most cardio exercises involve moves performed in front of the body, like tennis, swimming and boxing, but rowing is a great all-round workout that will relieve muscle fatigue from a tired back and neck, strengthen the back muscles and release held-in tension.

WORK IT!

To make your cardiovascular training effective, you should be prepared to workout at least 3–5 days a week for a duration of about 20 minutes. Incorporate interval training into your workout so you include "light" exercise with "hard" work where you intensify the heartbeat to 70–100% of the maximum heart rate.

JUMP IN

Swimming is one of the most effective fat-burning exercises you can do, as you are simultaneously working both the upper and lower body against the gravity of the water. It is great for toning flabby arms and legs and is achievable regardless of your overall level of fitness.

CLIMB EVERY MOUNTAIN

If you're going out for a weekend walk, choose a route with as many hills as possible. This will be a better workout for your heart and have a greater toning effect on flabby areas, particularly calves, thighs, and buttocks.

weight & resistance training

INCREASE YOUR METABOLISM

Strength-training exercises can raise the metabolic rate by about 30–50 calories per day. Over a three-month period, appropriate training will produce about 1.4 kg (3 lb) of muscle, which will boost your resting metabolic rate by about 7%.

WEIGHT TRAIN FOR BONE STRENGTH

Using free weights a couple of times a week for all-over strength training will significantly increase bone mineral density in the spine, which will help stop the vertebrae collapsing and decrease your chances of shrinkage.

HALT THE SHRINKING PROCESS

A strong straight back is key to keeping the height you had at 20. After the age of 40 we shrink around 1 cm (2/5 inch) every 10 years, so practice lying on your stomach with arms outstretched in front of you, and gently raise one arm for the count of 10 as you breathe out. Repeat 8 times per arm, alternating arms.

EASY DOES IT

Stretching is a gentle, easy exercise, so don't approach it as if you were racing through your workout. Be patient, use slow, deep movements, and never force it so you feel pain. Take your time and breathe naturally during your stretch, taking care never to hold your breath. If any stretch hurts you, eliminate it from your routine.

TOUCH YOUR TOES FOR ENERGY

For a quick shot of energy when you need it, bend over at the waist and hang your head down so that your hands touch your toes (or as near as you can get), and you're looking at your knees. Relax your upper body. Hold the position for several seconds and then slowly rise. This is a good morning starter that will also increase flexibility and help you align your posture.

GRAB A SET OF FREE WEIGHTS

Research has shown that free weights are more effective at building muscle tone than pushing against the resistance of machine weights. Plus you can do it at home or anywhere, any time.

INCREASE YOUR RANGE OF MOTION

Your stretch routine should address each section of the body and be dynamic, which means bringing a limb or muscle group through it's full range of motion slowly and smoothly.

INCREASE YOUR MOBILITY

Your joints can tighten and become thicker as you age but flexibility exercises can help increase the mobility. Bending, rotating and extending your joints prevents injury, so choose a good gentle stretching regime four or five days a week. Avoid any positions that can compress your vertebrae and put undue stress on your spine, however, such as vigorous forward or side twists.

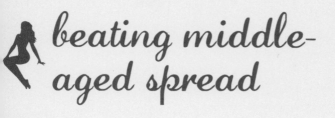

beating middle-aged spread

SORT OUT THE SOMATOPAUSE

Medical practitioners have defined the onset of middle-aged spread as the somatopause. Strenuous aerobic exercise has been shown to increase the production of hGH, the human growth hormone (which is responsible for this metabolic slow down), and which will help reverse classic middle-aged symptoms.

TUMMY TIGHTENER

Most of us spend far too many hours at work but when you are sitting at your desk, focus on tightening your tummy and your buttocks, holding for 20 seconds then relaxing for 20. Do this four times a day and you will notice the difference.

IT'S CRUNCH TIME

Abdominal crunches are the best way to tone all the muscle groups of the stomach, so don't neglect them. Regular exercises will strengthen the core muscle groups of the trunk, where all your body's movements originate. These muscles support your internal organs, aid in breathing, and work with the vertebrae to help your body bend and twist.

WAIST AWAY FOR OPTIMUM HEALTH

People prone to the "apple" shape who have a waist measurement of over 81 cm (32 inches) need to act now to avert potential danger of heart disease and diabetes. Losing even a small amount of weight, for example 10% of your body weight, will drastically reduce this dangerous layer of abdominal fat by 30%.

TONE THAT TUMMY

Shape up effortlessly with a Slendertone corset that stimulates muscles in the abdomen without you having to do a thing. Small pulsing contractions train muscles to be firmer and stronger, and regular use will reduce the size of waist.

DON'T LOVE YOUR LOVE HANDLES

Waist twists will help you target those unsightly love handles. It is a very low-impact exercise and a good precursor to abdominal crunch work. Stand with your feet flat on the floor and your fingertips touching the tops of your shoulders, and your arms bent at the elbow. Slowly twist the elbows, arms, and shoulders as if you are looking over your shoulder, following the movement of your upper body with your head, and keep your abdominal muscles tensed. Rotate to the other side.

TOP TUMMY TIP

A good one for your core muscles and to build arm muscle is to rest your tummy on an exercise ball and then walk out as far as you can so that the ball slowly moves towards your face. Keep your body as straight as possible, then walk back – five times a day is enough to see results.

TIGHTEN UP THE TORSO

Rollerblading and ice-skating are both good sports to keep the torso strong and toned. Using the arms to propel motion, the upper body has to stay strong to provide balance, so these activities work all the abdomen muscles in the process.

BUTTOCK AND BELLY LIFT

If you need a rest, this exercise involves lying flat on your back. Rest your ankles on an exercise ball; slowly raise your hips so that your body is in a straight line from the shoulders to the ankles. Hold for 30 seconds, then lower your hips. Repeat 10 times.

TONE THE TRUNK WITH PILATES

In middle age the build up of fat from a reduced metabolism usually forms around the waist and stomach. Pilates lessons focus on core stability exercises that target this trunk area to tone up waist and stomach and strengthen the lumbar region of the spine.

SIT UP AND WORK OUT

Just sitting on an exercise ball in front of the TV will provide benefits. Sit up straight, tighten your tummy muscles, and gently lift one foot off the floor at a time. Do this while watching your favourite TV show – multitasking is what we're good at!

buttocks & legs

IN-LINE FOR A PERT BUTT

For a workout that targets the backs of the thighs and the derrière more effectively than running or cycling try 30 minutes of in-line skating. It works the hip muscles and tightens up the gluteus maximus without too much hard work.

ANY TIME, ANY PLACE

Waiting in line at a bus stop or in the grocery store can be time well spent if you make an effort to clench your buttocks and hold for 30 seconds at a time. This will work the gluteus maximus muscles to firm up a flabby bottom and protect the lower spine.

TARGET THE INNER THIGH

Thighs that jiggle do not have to be a fact of life. Your hip adductors are those small muscles on the inner thighs that help you pull your legs together and apart. The most effective exercises for toning this area rely on the use of weights, bands or balls to provide resistance. Side-stepping quats and lunges are also effective.

LEG LUNGES FOR SHAPELY KNEES

If your knees are showing their age with crepey loose skin above the
kneecap, try incorporating leg lunges and squats into your workout
routine. Leg muscles build up quickly in just a few weeks, and the
lunges target the quad muscles at the front of the thigh, which support
the knee. Your hamstrings and glutes will also get a good workout.

A BETTER BACK END

You probably can't change your natural body shape but you can
tighten up a flabby derrière with regular lunging exercises. Stand up
straight, take a big step forward, and bend at the knee, then push back
up to a standing position.

THE BEST BOTTOM CLENCH

To keep your butt fit and taut, get in the habit of performing an easy
leg lift every time you clean your teeth. Hold onto the basin and lift
one leg out to the side and back, keeping the movement slow and
controlled with the foot flexed.

INCREASING SINGLE-LEG STRENGTH

Exercises to tone all the muscle groups of the legs will keep you
in good stead and allow you to maintain shapely legs; however
most exercises use conventional double-leg training which isn't as
effective as developing single-leg strength. Working one leg at a time
independently will help you with all your leg transitions (when you
move from one leg to another), which is when you walk, run, step,
reach or lunge.

SLIM THE SADDLEBAGS

To target the outer thigh area, which is prone to unsightly lumps
known as "saddlebags", stand up straight and lift your right leg out to
the side and then lower it. Remain erect without leaning, and repeat
10–12 times, before repeating with the other leg. For a more intensive
workout, strap on light ankle-weights.

attack bingo wings

SHOP AND TONE

When you're at the supermarket, forget the shopping cart and use a basket instead. This will help tone your arms, particularly if you do a few biceps curls while standing in the checkout line!

INTELLECTUAL WORKOUT

Another at-home exercise for your arms that will keep muscle tone firm and smooth is to clasp a heavy book in each hand then do arm lifts, from resting at your side to reaching out to shoulder level. While you've still got that heavy book in your hands, try lying flat on your back with your arms outstretched above your head. Now raise your arms until the book is above your head – try three sets of 10, three times a week.

WEIGHTS MAKE A DIFFERENCE

Make your power walk even more effective by carrying small hand weights with you. Walk purposefully using your arms to move you along, and arms and legs will benefit simultaneously.

WORK OUT WITH WEIGHTS

Cardiovascular work isn't enough to keep muscle tone built up as we get older. Regular arm exercises that use the same muscles repeatedly will result in beautifully contoured arms, and a faster metabolism, as muscle burns more calories than fat.

PLAY TENNIS FOR TRICEPS TONING

The triceps muscles at the back of the arms make-up two-thirds of the arm's size so strengthening this hard-to-reach area will make a noticeable improvement to your arms' shape. Practising your overhead swing can really help with toning, as can triceps dips and kickbacks.

EVERYDAY ARM DIPS

No one wants bingo wings, as they are the surest sign of middle-age. To make sure your upper arms are never an embarrassment, do triceps dips whenever you can – all you need is a chair!

BIG BALL PRESS-UPS

You will need to concentrate to stop yourself from falling off when you start doing push-ups on an exercise ball, but this manoeuver will make a big difference. Three sets of 10, three times a week, is all you need to reduce flabby bingo wings and tone up core muscles.

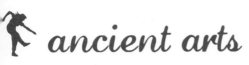 ancient arts

STAND ON YOUR HEAD

Get into the habit of standing on your head first thing in the morning.
In yoga this pose is called the "king of asanas" because of the
rejuvenating affect it has on just about every body cell. It is thought
to slow down the ageing process dramatically.

STRENGTHEN YOUR SPINE

The shoulder stand is a challenging yoga pose that has great benefits
for the whole body. It's important to warm up before going into it,
but it boosts circulation, stimulates the thyroid gland, and strengthens
the shoulders, arms and upper back.

HOLD DOWNWARD DOG

Take a yoga lesson to bring together the body, mind and spirit into
an integrated whole. The physical benefits are increased flexibility,
strength and stamina, as well as an inner sense of wellbeing, positivity
and clarity.

MEDITATION IN MOTION

The ancient Chinese art of tai chi is a non-competitive type of exercise
that has physical as well as mental benefits. It is used to reduce stress
and to increase energy and general feelings of wellbeing.

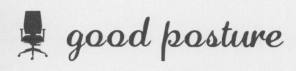 *good posture*

GAIN HEIGHT WITH PILATES

Pilates exercises help maintain a straight, strong spine, and keeping the spine aligned correctly in a controlled way will help prevent the spine from curving. To stay in alignment, imagine a piece of string that runs vertically through your spine and through the top of your head.

I MUST, I MUST IMPROVE MY BUST

Improved posture can create the illusion of a bigger chest. Make a conscious effort to stand up straight, as an erect spine naturally lifts the ribcage and enables the breasts to sit more pertly on the chest. Seek assistance from a chiropractor if you can't improve your posture on your own.

SIT PRETTY TO AVOID NECK PAIN

Common causes of neck pain are the natural degeneration of the spine and poor posture. Prevent pain by maintaining good posture when you are sitting for long periods. Avoid performing tasks that can strain the neck, such as reading or knitting for prolonged periods. Change your position periodically, and avoid napping in chairs as the neck can cramp uncomfortably.

AVOID OLD-AGE SLUMP

When meeting new people be aware of standing upright and tucking your buttocks in. Avoid slouching, slumping and leaning against walls to prop yourself up. Take your hands out of your pockets, and straighten rounded shoulders. Nothing is more ageing than a hunched back and poor posture.

RELAX YOUR SHOULDERS

Tension, stress and anxiety all make us scrunch our shoulders up, giving us the appearance of a hunchback as well as head and neck aches. Remind yourself to push your shoulders back and down, and relax the muscles for better posture.

CHOOSE AN ERGONOMIC CHAIR

Sitting in an ergonomically designed chair while you work will reduce the damage of hunched shoulders and a bad back, but you should still have a regular spinal stretch and roll your head from side to side to help keep your back straight and strong.

WALK TALL THE ALEXANDER WAY

Good posture is one of the best and easiest ways to defy age. The Alexander Technique teaches you to stand, sit, and walk in perfect alignment, as well as improving stamina and flexibility.

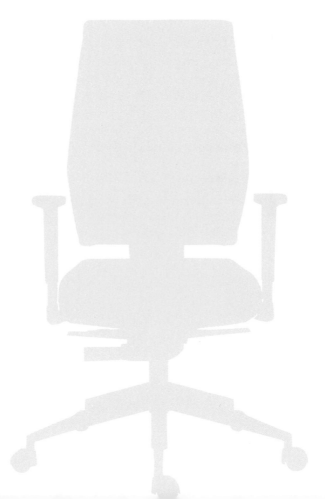

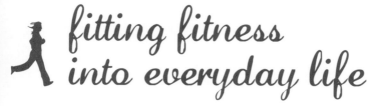

fitting fitness into everyday life

KEEP MOVING

Every day think of something you can do to get the blood pumping. Always take the most energetic option if you have a choice: walk up stairs instead of taking the elevator, and even walk up escalators if you can. Take a bike ride instead of using the car for short distances, or park the car some distance away and walk the remaining way to your destination.

SUPPORT YOUR TEAM

If your children play for a soccer team, volunteer to be a "linesman". Running up and down the touchline for an hour is great exercise, and because you'll be cheering them on at the same time you won't even notice how much running you're doing. Take every opportunity you have to exercise with your kids or grandkids – not only will it help your health but it will also set good habits and you'll be a role model for them.

FORGET TO SIT DOWN

Try to do your ordinary tasks while standing or walking around as this will help you avoid spending long periods of time sitting, which can lead to an increased risk of thrombosis and swollen ankles. For example, every time the phone rings, stand up and walk around to talk.

WORK IT OUT

Get outside in the garden and do some physical digging, raking or shovelling soil. Research has shown that an afternoon spent working in the garden uses as much energy as casual cycling or walking, and the whole body gets a workout as you are lifting, stretching and occasionally weightlifting.

DON'T LIKE THE GYM, DON'T GO!

If you find the tedium of the treadmill boring, find some other aerobic exercise that is fun and challenging. Tennis, salsa dancing, fencing, or ballet will all increase your heartbeat, keep you fit and supple, and are good social opportunities, plus they can be done long into your later years.

THE JOY OF BIKES

Rediscover the pleasure of bicycling to and from stores. Short hops will tone up legs and calves, and if you really start to enjoy it you can start muddy mountain biking, which will improve all-over fitness and bring a rosy glow to your skin.

HANG IT HIGH

If you hang your washing outside on the line, make sure the line is high above your head. Endless reaching up to pin the clothes will give your spine a thorough stretch and stop you hunching. Make the most of other chores around the house, too, such as getting a good upper-body workout from washing your car or engaging in vigorous spring cleaning.

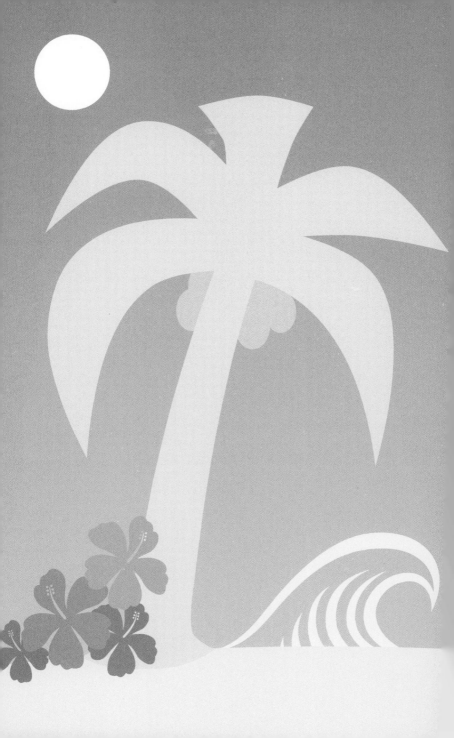

Special Occasions

FROM TRAVEL BEAUTY to big nights out, this section offers indispensable tips on beauty for special occasions, including during pregnancy and adjusting for a change of seasons. In addition, help is on hand for such emergency situations as tanning mistakes, overplucked brows, angry-looking blemishes and red eyes.

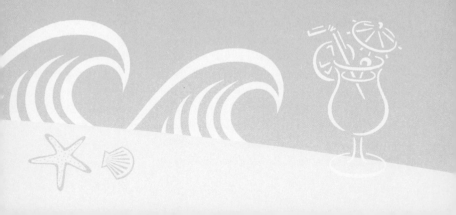

❶ beauty emergencies

DIMINISH UNDER-EYE BAGS
For a great solution to firm up under-eye bags and wrinkles, follow
the A-list and invest in some haemorrhoid cream, which firms up and
tightens skin in delicate areas.

TEST YOUR IODINE
If you have coarse hair, dry skin and suffer from tiredness, you may
be experiencing low iodine levels. Seafood and seaweed are the best
sources, or ask your doctor for an iodine test if you're really worried.

START SMALL
If you suffer eyeshadow creasing, use a small eyeshadow brush with a
very small amount of colour and apply in layers to avoid over-doing it.
Avoid cream shadows, which have a greater tendency to crease.

DON'T BE A RED-RIMMED SPECTACLE
Lack of vitamin C can lead to styes and inflammation and redness
of the rims and whites of the eyes. Rich sources are citrus fruits and
juices, kiwis, strawberries, broccoli and potatoes.

POWDER IT OUT
As a quick solution to greasy or oily hair, particularly around the
forehead, a dab of translucent powder along the hairline can soak up
excess moisture and tide you over until you hit the shower.

GLOSS OVER EMERGENCIES
Always keep an emergency lip gloss in your handbag. For those
sudden meetings or dates, a subtly coloured gloss is the perfect way to
dress up your mouth without going over the top.

ROSY CHEEKS
When you don't have enough time to apply make-up, but you don't
want to be seen naked-faced, rosy up your cheeks with a quick slick of
cream blusher for a naturally beautiful glow.

TURN ON THE NUDES

To even out self-tan streaks or blotches on the face, use a tinted moisturizer, but avoid any cheek colour or bronzer – instead choose neutral eye and lip colours so that your look is as fresh as possible and you aren't drawing attention to the face.

ICE THOSE COLD SORES

If you feel the tingling sensation of a cold sore, treat the area with ice immediately, which can help reduce the inflammation around the site and stop the sore from developing. Once the sore has erupted, dab it with salt and lemon.

BIG SQUEEZE

You've squeezed a spot and it's red and inflamed. Now what? Apply antibacterial ointment and wait for the area to dry. Then apply concealer to the red area and over the base of the spot. Avoid covering up a spot with loose powder before it's dry as the powder can cause the spot to turn crusty – wait until the blemish has stopped weeping first.

DE-PUFF UNDER-EYE BAGS

If you wake up in the morning with puffy, swollen eyes, apply a gel-based under-eye product to de-puff the tender skin around your eyes, followed by a cool compress – eye masks, which can be kept in the fridge overnight, are a great choice.

HIDE TANNING MISTAKES

If you're out and about in the evening, a light-reflecting product will help even out skin tone and disguise any major streaks caused by badly applied self-tan.

GET SALTY

Reduce your chances of infection in cuts and broken skin using salt to cleanse and detoxify small wounds. Or sprinkle a pinch of turmeric onto cuts to boost the skin's natural healing process. To stop bleeding from a shaving nick, use a styptic pencil but if you don't have one, try a tiny dab of anti-perspirant, alcohol or peroxide.

GLOW EVEN WHEN YOU'RE LOW

Apply bronzer lightly across your forehead and under your cheekbones to add a healthy sheen to hungover or over-tired skin, which will help you feel brighter and will stop everyone at work commenting on how tired you look.

HORROR HAIR COLOUR

If you hate your colour, do not ever try to correct it yourself with an at-home dye or go to an alternative hairdresser. Immediately return to the original stylist, tell them you are unhappy and ask if they can remedy the situation. They prefer happy clients, so will usually comply, free of charge, and you won't be throwing good money after bad.

WATER IT WELL

If your skin looks pale and your eyes dull, this could be the first signs of dehydration, and simply topping up your water levels could give your looks a boost.

PENCIL IT IN

To correct over-plucked eyebrows, choose an eyebrow pencil as close to your brow colour as possible and lightly pencil in, following your natural line. Use short pencil strokes, then brush out your brow to soften the line.

PRIME SKIN WITH POST-LUNCH POWDER

After lunch the skin on your face can often become shiny and greasy. Dust on an oil-free powder to cut out the shine, but don't go overboard; just stick to a thin layer and reapply the powder later if necessary.

FIX UP A SHAKY FOUNDATION

Like energy levels, foundation can flag by four O' clock in the afternoon, but a five-minute bathroom touch-up will do the trick. First, blot your face to get rid of excess oil and then blend in foundation that has creased using a clean make-up sponge. Dust translucent powder all over and swipe on a subtle blush and lipstick.

TRY THE TOOTHPASTE TRICK

If you suddenly find you have a spot the night before a big party or interview, apply toothpaste to it overnight, which will help dry out the skin and reduce redness around the area.

SMALL IS BEAUTIFUL

Cover a problem spot with a small, pointy brush dipped in concealer and paint it out – a tiny brush allows you to target the blemish without making the cover-up attempt obvious. Choose a brush with a lid so you can retouch the spot easily.

HAVE A CUPPA FOR PUFFY EYES

For soothing and reducing puffiness in tired, swollen eyes, soak a couple of tea bags in warm water. Squeeze them until just damp and rest for ten minutes with the tea bags on closed eyes. Tea's natural antioxidant properties will get to work on your problem.

WIPE UP AFTER WORKOUTS

Even if you don't feel like you've sweated much during exercise, chances are your skin has evaporated more moisture. For a quick fix post-exercise, when you don't have time for a full shower, use cleansing wipes to remove sweat and oil. Clean skin will reduce the chance of blemishes and keep the pores clear.

TAKE THE SPONGE

If there's one thing you should carry with you in case of beauty emergencies, it's a packet of clean cosmetic sponges, which can be used to smooth out or reapply foundation, blend creased eyeshadow and blend streaky areas.

LIP UP YOUR CHEEKS

When you're caught looking pale or tired with nothing on you but a lipstick, use a few dabs on your cheeks, blended in with fingers, to give yourself a healthy glow.

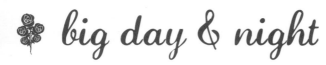# big day & night

FIRST THINGS FIRST

For big nights out you want your eye make-up to last until the wee hours. To provide a good base, first apply foundation on your eyelids only, and then apply your eyeshadow. When done, lightly mist water over your eyes to set. Then apply the rest of your foundation and make-up as usual.

GO WARM ON BRIDAL LIPS

Brides should choose a lip colour in a warm, fairly bright shade. Roses, pinks and reds look great in photos and keep teeth and wedding whites looking clean and fresh.

BE LAVISH WITH LASHES

Create lush lashes by using an eyelash curler and applying two thin coats of lengthening mascara. Don't overwhelm your lashes with too many coats, especially if your big moment is in the daytime, because your lashes can look clumpy and there's more chance of fall-out. Waterproof mascara is longlasting and won't run if you shed a few tears of joy.

GET A PROFESSIONAL LOOK

Head to your nearest make-up counter or boutique for a special consultation. Not only will they be able to show you great colours, but they'll also give you tips on techniques and insider tricks as well. Sometimes high-profile make-up artists make store visits so keep an eye out for any advertisement giving dates and times for these free events.

UP-DO HAIR-DO

For a wedding day, black-tie event or other formal occasion, try a sleek sophisticated chignon. Visit your hairdresser for a trial run first to see how it will look and whether it will suit your dress. Your stylist will be able to advise on using hairpieces and aids to achieve the look you want.

GO WARM ON CHEEKS

For wedding days, when you naturally want to emphasize your youth
and beauty, choose a warm, flattering cheek colour in a pinky peach
or rose, which will look like a natural extension of your skin tone.
Focus on the rounded parts of the cheek and blend the blush back and
up toward your hairline.

TEST WHAT LOOKS BEST

Always try at least one test-run of what you'd like to look like on your
big day – with full dress, hair and make-up. Do it a few weeks before
the big event and time yourself so that you know to leave enough time
on the day itself. For make-up, think about what time of day you want
to make your best impression, and don't be afraid to change your
look if the occasion runs from day into evening, adding some darker
colours or sparkle if you are going to be dancing later on.

DON'T FOLLOW FASHION

Don't get too trendy with your eye make-up on your wedding day. You
may think that sparkly eyeliner is a good idea today, but chances are
you'll look back at the pictures years from now and regret it. Keep it
natural and fresh and be wary of using a make-up artist who doesn't
know you well – they could make your look too strong or too pale for
you, and you'll spend needless time retouching your face.

AVOID THE BURN

Don't get too much sun before a big event. Sunburns, peeling skin
and tan lines can sabotage your special day because they're difficult to
cover up completely.

KEEP YOUR FACE ON

Give your foundation staying power by using a gel foundation primer
before you apply your make-up. Add a light dusting of loose powder
to prevent any unwanted shine.

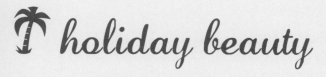 holiday beauty

STAY ABOVE THE CUT

Before you go on a beach holiday, take a trip to the hairdresser for a pre-holiday trim. Damaged ends will only get worse when exposed to the drying effects of sun, salt and chlorine, so make sure you set off with your hair in tiptop form.

CARRY ON CAMPING

Space is at a premium in a tent so you won't want to take your usual bottles of cleanser and toner. Extra-mild baby wipes are a brilliant substitute, even for removing stubborn mascara, and can be helpful for many other cleaning tasks.

BE A GLOSS ADJUSTER

Before you go away, protect your hair using a semi-permanent gloss colour treatment, which will not only make you feel great but also adds a layer of protection to your hair, preventing it from moisture loss. To really bolster hair health, treat yourself to a deep-conditioning treatment, either using a rich cream mask or a treatment oil to boost moisture and gleam.

PLAIT IT UP

If you have long hair, consider putting it into a plait when you're on the beach or by the pool – this will reduce the amount of hair (especially ends) which are in contact with the sun's damaging rays and help your hair stay looking healthy.

PREVENT BITES WITH COAL TAR

Using coal tar soap to wash yourself in the bath or shower can help keep biting insects at bay, so you don't arrive home from your holiday covered in bites and itchy marks.

STROLL IN THE SEA

Give your bum and thighs a workout by strolling in water that's at least knee deep. It will keep you cool in the sun and, because you're working against resistance, help tone up your legs and bottom.

CURL AND DYE

Have your lashes curled and dyed before you jet off to the beach and you won't have to worry about waterproof mascara or panda eyes. Tints have the added bonus of swelling your lashes, making them appear thicker.

SKI AWAY TO BEAUTY

Cold mountain air and high altitudes can wreak havoc with moisture levels, so be sure to drink as much water as you can. Avoid astringents or clay face masks, which are drying. Instead of foundation, cover blemishes and red areas with concealer and use a copious amount of sunblock, paying particular attention to the hairline and ears.

BE SHORE-FOOTED

Walking on sand is one of the best ways to naturally exfoliate your feet and reduce foot tension, as the hard grains give you a massage and pedicure at the same time!

PRICKLY PAIR

If you find yourself suffering from prickly heat – small red bumps on the skin that itch severely – wear natural fibres like cotton and linen, and don't be tempted to scratch, which will make it worse. Products containing salicylic acid can help.

VISIT AN EXPERT

If your hair has suffered while you were away, pay a trip to your hairdresser as soon as you get back for a quick trim to remove damaged ends. That way, the damage and splits won't spread up the hair shafts.

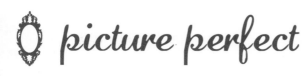

picture perfect

SIGH AWAY CHINS, LOOK BLINKS AWAY
To avoid double chins in photographs, take a deep breath just before
the shutter goes down and sigh out as you smile or pose, which will
tighten the area under the chin and avoid it sagging. If you tend to blink
in photos, look down or to the side, and just before the photographer is
ready to take the shot, move your eyes back to the camera.

FIND AN INTERESTING ANGLE
Look at photos of yourself that you like and try to replicate your
position in the future. Many people look better with their head
slightly angled to the side than straight on.

USE CONTRAST
Photography, especially if there's a flash involved, can wash out pale
colours. To prepare for important photographs, consider putting on a
little more make-up than normal to ensure you look your best.

AVOID FROSTING
For photos, never make the mistake of wearing a lipstick that is too
neutral or frosted. These colours can leave you looking pale or tired
and will wash out your face.

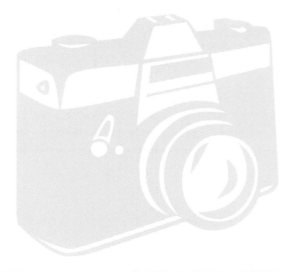

SIMMER ON THE SHIMMER

Don't get carried away with shimmer highlighters. In photos, these can give you an unflattering and highly reflective shine, which may look very overdone. Aim for subtlety.

GET SIDEWAYS

In groups, don't be the one caught in the middle with both your arms around the others, which can make you look wider as you are facing the camera straight on. Instead, use one arm around another person and keep the other arm low.

SIDE ON

For a slimming standing pose, copy the celebrities and hold your body at a three-quarter pose with one foot in front of the other and with your arms held away from your body – this will minimize the amount of space your body takes up and make your extremities look leaner. Stand tall with the shoulders back. At the moment before the picture is taken, tuck your bottom in slightly – this thrusts the hips out a little and makes your torso look longer.

DON'T DRESS TO IMPRESS

Don't use a heavy pressed powder to set your foundation if you want to look your best in photographs. Too much powder can leave your skin looking chalky and dull.

GO YELLOW IN A FLASH

Foundations with slightly yellow undertones work best with flash photography, so be careful with rose tones which can look harsh and make you appear red in the face.

BE EDGY

For sitting photographs, move to the edge of your chair so your thighs drop down rather than spread out and look larger than they actually are.

THINGS ARE LOOKING UP

If someone is taking a shot of your face and you want your cheeks to look slimmer, ask them to take it from above you. Looking up at the camera will widen your eyes and narrow your cheeks. A quick trick to avoid the appearance of a double chin is to touch your tongue to the roof of your mouth.

DON'T BE BROWBEATEN

Remember that photos increase contrast, so don't use dark shadows or pencils to define your brows, as this may leave you looking stern rather than stunning. Likewise too much kohl eyeliner and smoky eyeshadows can create dark pools in the eye area, making your eyes appear much more deeply set.

THE LOWDOWN ON LOOKING GOOD

Unless you're super tall, never let anyone take a full-length photo of you from eye level, as this will shorten your legs. Ask them to squat on the ground and aim up for a more flattering leg-lengthening angle.

☼ seasonal beauty

BEWARE OF SPOTS

Spots are more common in spring than winter, as the skin begins to produce the oils it has been lacking over the dry winter months. Cleanse day and night and switch your moisturizer to a light formula.

STEAM AHEAD

Once a week during the spring months treat your facial skin to at-home herbal steam therapy using Ayurvedic powders or homemade versions by steeping garden herbs in boiling water. This will help to rejuvenate the skin's natural detox process.

PREPARE TO BARE

It's not just the skin on your face which needs attention in spring. Most likely, your body has been covered up during the winter months, so make sure you welcome it back to exposure with all-over exfoliation and moisturization.

LESS IS MORE IN SUMMERTIME

If you change one thing with the seasons, make it your base. Winter foundation will look dull and heavy in the summer, when the light is brighter and your skin is a different colour. Switch to a lighter formula, a tinted moisturizer or just use concealer and a sunscreen.

HIT THE WATER BOTTLE

Drink lots of water throughout the day during summer months, not only to replenish moisture lost to the heat and sweat, but also to help flush toxins out of the body and keep skin looking clear and lustrous. Herb or spice teas, made with skin-enhancing ingredients, offer added therapeutic benefits.

BEAT THE OIL

The sun can increase sebum production, causing your skin to look oily on occasion. When the oil combines with dirt and sweat, pores get clogged. In summer, you must be meticulous about your cleansing routine, morning and night, especially if you're using sun-blocking creams. If you really suffer from oily skin, avoid night-time moisturizers to give your skin a break.

GET RICH QUICK

Use a rich daily moisturizer to keep skin plumped up and well oiled during winter months when it can often become dry and dull. This will help it retain a healthy glow. If possible, avoid AHAs, retinol products and strong exfoliators that strip away your skin in winter and look for enriching ingredients such as vitamin E, amino acids, hyaluronic acid that will quench dry skin.

LIGHTEN YOUR SCENTS

Choose a light formula of fragrance for the summer months – an eau de toilette or a body spritz in the floral or ozonic family is more refreshing and suitable than the autumnal woody and spicy chypre and fougère fragrances.

TAKE A WALK ON THE MILD SIDE

If you want to enjoy the sun, go easy on spicy and very sour foods, like chilli, lime and vinegar, which may increase skin's reactivity to sunlight and cause irritation. Stick to milder foods with high water content instead.

MILK IT

Milk has cooling properties, which supply nutrients to the skin and keep it from drying out by assisting in forming a protective layer against water loss. Drink a glass of milk every day in hot weather, or choose cleansers and moisturizers with milk added.

MASK THE PROBLEM

Once a week during summer, use a face mask derived from fruit to help rebalance and rejuvenate summer skin, removing excess oils without drying. Avocado, cucumber and papaya are all great fruit mask choices.

DEVOTE TIME TO YOUR DECOLLETAGE

The skin on your chest and neck is almost as delicate as that on your face, but it's easily forgotten in the autumn, when you're likely to start covering up more. Apply a moisturizer at night on your neck, ears and collarbone area, as well as your face to keep it toned.

COME ON STRONG

Dull colours in winter mean thickening up make-up looks great. Go for black rather than the beiges and browns of summer, and risk metallic shades and darker lips, which will smoulder in winter's flatter light.

BE CLUED UP ABOUT CLEANSERS

Autumn brings with it colder weather, which means the oils the skin has been producing liberally throughout the warmth of the summer begin to fade. Make sure autumn cleansers are free from detergents which could strip the skin of moisture.

A COMPACT SOLUTION

Even dry skins can shine in the summer. Take a powder compact with you at all times to correct the extra shine and you may even be able to forgo foundation or tinted moisturizer entirely. Fight bacteria by using a make-up brush for dabbing on the powder, rather than the pad applicator that comes with the compact.

GO YELLOW

Be aware that summer light has more yellow tones to it than winter's grey. Choose your tones carefully and make sure you check your make-up in daylight before you venture out. Look out for sallow areas around eyes and neck.

BE A PLUM FAIRY

Instead of immediately opting for dark colours in the autumn, step slowly into winter with deep berry colours, plums and slate greys, which blend with summer skin and brighten dark autumn nights. Simply choosing a different shade of lipstick can be enough to direct your look toward the new season.

WAKE UP WITH WATER AND LEMON

This Chinese herbal remedy is a sure-fire method of energizing your body. It will detox your entire system, including the liver and gall bladder, which means your body will be able to clean the blood faster to rid itself of the toxins responsible for poor skin. Simply add a few slices of fresh lemon or the juice of half a lemon to a cup of hot water and drink it.

DON'T BE HOT TO TROT

The thought of a long, hot bath on a cold, winter day can be appealing, but over-exposure to hot water can dry skin out even more. Keep baths or showers short, limit them to one per day and use warm, not hot, water.

AIM FOR SPF8

Unless you're skiing, you don't need a high SPF during the winter, when the sunlight is weaker. Change down from an SPF 15 to an 8 to give your skin a chance to absorb vitamin D and avoid developing sensitivity to the chemicals in sunscreens.

PLAY INDOOR BOWLS

To combat the drying effects of central heating, place houseplants in your home and office (and water or mist them frequently). For an instant humidifier in the bedroom, place a bowl of water near a radiator or heat source to keep moisture levels high in the room and aid respiration overnight.

GO MILD

Throw away soap, which can irritate drier skin, and switch to a milder, gentler cleanser for face and body. Soap can irritate and exacerbate dry skin conditions. Instead of rubbing yourself dry, pat to remove excess moisture.

NO TIME TO CHAP

Chapped lips are often the most noticeable problem when it comes to dryness in the winter. Use a highly moisturizing lip balm, which provides a protective barrier, with vitamin E for good elasticity.

SCRUB UP WELL

Exfoliate once a week to remove dead skin cells and allow the skin to absorb extra moisture, which is lost from the skin's lower layers during winter because of harsher, cooler temperatures. It will help your skin stay pink and glowing rather than grey and dull.

yummy mummies

BANISH BRUISES WITH MARIGOLD

Pregnant skin is more prone to bruising. Make a bruise-busting
infusion with a handful of marigold (calendula officianalis) flowers
and 300 ml (½ pint) of boiled water. Steep for five minutes,
allow to cool, then wipe the bruised area. Arnica cream is a good
homeopathic alternative.

CHOOSE CREAM CAREFULLY

The best creams to prevent stretch marks from occurring are those
that contain collagen and elastin, which help regenerate the skin's
lower layers and reduce the chances of it being stretched and scarred.

FEED HUNGRY SKIN

The turnover of skin cells is accelerated during pregnancy as the
metabolic rate increases, so make sure you nourish and moisturize
more than normal to keep skin looking healthy. Concentrate on areas
that expand, like the breasts and abdomen. Choose moisturizers that
are as pure as possible, such as cocoa butter, as everything you put on
your skin has a chance of being absorbed into the bloodstream.

E-RASE STRETCH MARKS

Use vitamin E cream on stretch marks, massaging it into delicate
or affected areas once or twice a day to make them less visible
and to prevent others appearing in the first place.

BE PATIENT WITH PIGMENT CHANGES

Some women suffer marked pigment changes on their face in
pregnancy – called chloasma – because of hormonal changes.
If you suffer from this, avoid the sun (which makes it worse)
and use make-up to even out your skin tone. Your complexion
should revert to normal a few months after the baby is born.

MASSAGE YOUR BUMP

Skin is under a great deal of pressure during pregnancy, with a lot of stretching to do, especially in the abdominal area. Massaging your bump with oil, cream or gel will keep skin supple and elastic, and boost circulation. This will also provide relief if you suffer from an itchy belly.

CHANGE PRODUCTS

When you're pregnant, hormones cause changes and sensitivity in your natural skin and hair, so reconsider the suitability of your normal products, which may not be the best to use at this time.

LOVE YOUR CURVES

Instead of worrying about your growing curves, make the most of them with softer hair and make-up for a more feminine look. It's only nine months, after all, and the sooner you accept your new curves, the more you'll enjoy them!

FAKE TAN MAKES MARKS FAINT

Fake tan will help conceal stretch marks by colouring the skin and minimizing their visibility. This trick is especially good for silvery pink marks. Real tanning, however, makes stretchmarks more obvious, so stay out of the sun.

FEED YOUR FEET

Feet can get tired and swollen in pregnancy as the body copes with high levels of blood and fluid circulating in the body. A refreshing foot gel with menthol will really pep you up at the end of a long day, especially if you rest with your feet up.

SWIM WELL AS YOU SWELL

Swimming is one of the best exercises for pregnancy because all the body is supported, but chlorine and chemicals can strip skin of moisture and leave it feeling dull and dry. Make sure you use rich body lotions to counteract the drying effects.

STAND TALL

With all the changes in weight and gravity that your body goes
through as part of a normal pregnancy, your back may tend to slouch.
Try to keep your hips in line with your shoulders rather than pushing
them forward as you stand or walk. Good posture will not only help
you look taller and less dumpy but will evenly distribute the strain of
the added baby weight.

RETREAT FROM RETIN-A

Increased androgen levels make women more prone to blemishes
during the first three months of pregnancy, but you should avoid
using acne medications which may cause harm to the developing
foetus. These include vitamin A-derivative lotions such as Accutane
and Retin-A.

GO VEGGIE

Any hair colouring process should avoid touching the skin and scalp
to prevent the absorption of chemicals into the bloodstream during
pregnancy. To be safe, opt for highlights and streaks which do not
touch the scalp, instead of all-over colour. Rather than your usual
bleach or ammonia highlights while pregnant, ask for vegetable dyes
or use henna, which do not contain chemicals.

DON'T REACH OILING POINT

If your skin suffers from oiliness during pregnancy, particularly on
your face, make sure your cleansers, moisturizers and suncreams are
labelled as non-comedogenic (not pore-blocking) and non-acnegenic
(not spot-causing).

EXTEND YOUR EXFOLIATION

Skin regenerates itself more quickly during pregnancy, which means
dead skin cells are more likely to build up on the surface, causing
dullness and spots. Thoroughly cleanse your face morning and night
and use a gentle exfoliator on the face and body two or three times a
week to keep skin soft, clear and uncongested.

EXTREMITIES NEED EXTRA CARE

Skin on the hands, feet, lower legs and arms is often neglected by the circulation system during pregnancy, as the body concentrates on the growing baby. Gentle exercises and massage can help encourage blood flow to the area to counteract dryness and tingling sensations.

FACE UP TO THE NEW YOU

Many women's face shapes change during pregnancy, becoming fuller and more rounded. Rather than lamenting it, ask your hairdresser to suggest subtle changes to your hair to flatter your new look – straight, shoulder-length hair can help slim cheeks, for example.

CUT DOWN ON CHEMICALS

Instead of using chemical products or straighteners to create a smooth look, which might affect the baby, dry your hair straight using a straightening balm, a natural bristle brush and a nozzled hairdryer. Alternatively, try a light-hold gel to keep natural curls tamed.

BABY KNOWS BEST

Mild baby products are suitable for sensitive skin that is going through hormonal upheavals, so raid your child's supply of baby oil, shampoo and talcum powder. Choose unscented varieties.

HEAD FOR A SCARF

Long hair can seem extra hot and bothersome when you're pregnant or in care of a small babe. Keeping locks held back with a fashionable hairband or scarf will allow you to go about your daily jobs in comfort without compromising your sex appeal.

COUNT TO THREE

Most doctors and hair stylists recommend not submitting your hair to any chemical processes during the first three months of pregnancy because of extra sensitivity to chemical fumes. This includes colouring, perming or chemical straightening. Even after this, always seek professional advice, as there is ongoing debate as to whether the processes are safe for the baby. To make safe hair colour changes, try a hair wand, gel or mascara, which give a temporary non-toxic colour highlight that only lasts as long as your next wash.

IT'S HARD NOT TO DRY

Breastfeeding can make hair very dry, as the body directs most of its nutrients towards the baby. It should return to normal once you stop, but an extra-moisturizing shampoo and deep conditioner will help until then.

BEWARE OF THE BARE

One of the biggest beauty mistakes pregnant women make is abandoning cosmetics entirely. Instead, lightly make-up eyes and lips to help you feel like a natural beauty. Because of the increased bloodflow in the body, cheeks often become red and blotchy. Cover them up with a natural-looking foundation or concealer and keep them well moisturized to prevent dry and flaky patches.

IT MAKES SCENTS

Make the most of your heightened sense of smell and give yourself a lift by spritzing on a clean, fresh scent. Choose a light floral or ozonic fragrance that won't overpower you or make you feel nauseous.

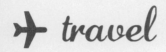 *travel*

BE A WATER BABY
For every hour onboard a flight, you can lose 100 ml (3½ fl oz)
of water from your skin. Keep hydrated by drinking at least 250 ml
(8½ fl oz) of water every hour and moisturize your face and body well
before flying.

SAFE LANDINGS
Post-flight skin is usually tired and dehydrated, so using lots of
make-up to make yourself look better won't help. Instead, apply
moisturizer and smudge cheeks with colour-enhancing cream blush or
gel bronzer. Use an oil or moisturizer containing vitamin E, which will
help beat sagginess and give skin a plumper feel.

USE A FACE TREATMENT
Instead of accepting that flying will make your skin look bad, fight off
dullness by using a face treatment while you're on board, particularly
on your cheeks, which are often the first areas to show telltale signs of
dehydration like fine lines.

TRAVEL WITH A TINT
Tinted moisturizer is an excellent product for travelling. Not only
is it easy to transport and apply, but it can work equally well as a
moisturizer, foundation and SPF all in one. It's also less drying than
many foundations, which is a must for dehydrated skin.

PACK IN THE BOX
Instead of carrying a handful of lipsticks with you on holiday, invest
in a pill case and fill the sections with different lip shades. Not only
have you created your own lip palette, you'll also be able to leave the
rest at home, preventing heat damage.

SLEEP IN THE CLOUDS

The best thing you can do on a plane is to sleep as much as you can. Get comfortable by using a neck pillow, as this area of the body is the one most prone to stiffness after a flight. Invest in an eye mask and ear plugs to block out excess light and noise, whatever the distractions.

WAKE YOURSELF UP

Humidity is usually less than 20% in airplanes. To freshen dehydrated skin and eyes on longhaul flights, splash your face with cold water and apply plenty of light, non-clogging moisturizer and an eye cream. This will tone the skin and enliven puffy eyes. Spritzing the face with a rosewater atomizer during the flight will also help keep skin supple and soft.

GLOSS IT UP

If you're travelling to warmer climes, lipstick sometimes seems too chalky or heavy. Instead, take a lipliner and lip gloss in your handbag. Line lightly or colour in the whole lip for an instant natural boost that will stay on your lips for hours.

MULTITASK YOUR MAKE-UP

Triple crayons and multi-use products like lip and cheek stains are great for travelling because you can apply them on the go with fingers for a quick boost and they take up precious little space in your handbag. Vaseline also makes a great moisturizer, lip balm, highlighter and first-aid salve.

USE UP YOUR FREEBIES

Take any extra free trial-size products from magazines or beauty counters with you. Don't be afraid to ask for samples at beauty counters – in addition to providing good miniature-sizes for travelling and weekends away, it will enable you to try out a product first before investing in a costly purchase for the full-size item.

BE BOLD WITH BRONZER

Travelling often makes skin look tired and dull. Bronzer is a great all-round product for warming up pale skin and gives you a glow. It can also be used as a blush or eyeshadow for a more grown-up look.

FLEX THE FEET

For a quick exercise during a train, car or plane journey where you will be stationary for some time, stand on one foot and bend the other behind you, grasping the ankle in your hand. Now flex and unflex your foot – this will keep the blood flowing and help prevent thrombosis and pins and needles.

DON'T TOIL WITH YOUR TOILETRIES

Decant your everyday supplies into plastic bottles to take with you – this will avoid any glass breakages and ensure that your toiletry kit is user-friendly and lightweight.

VANITY CASE

Keep everything at home that you can, taking only the essentials with you. Look for multiple-use products, such as cleansers that double as moisturizers, body lotions that are also formulated for hair conditioning and shea butter balm that conditions nails, hands and lips. A palette of lip, eye and cheek colours will take up much less space than individual products.

BRIGHTEN UP

To instantly enliven a tired face, blend a bit of illuminizer or radiance booster over the centre of the chin, the bridge of the nose and the middle of the forehead, which will help give the appearance of a natural, vital glow. If your neck or shoulders are bare, add a little there, too.

SUNSHINE INCREASES THE GREASE

Hot summer sunshine can increase sweat production and make your scalp look and feel much greasier. To counteract this problem, try more frequent washing with a small amount of shampoo, and use a much lighter conditioner.

DETOX POLLUTED HAIR

In the summer months there are higher levels of humidity and pollution in the air, so hair should be washed and conditioned more frequently using a good detox shampoo which will clean the hair gently without stripping away natural oils.

SUNLIGHT DAMAGES PRODUCTS

Keep conditioners and styling products away from the beach, as they need to be kept in a cool, shady place. Exposure to strong sunlight will destroy some of the active ingredients that make these hair products work.

REMEDY SCARECROW HAIR

A week of sun, salt water and chlorine will all play havoc with your hair, so spend one day with your hair covered in an intensive conditioner, slicked back and covered with a fashionable Pucci- or Hermes-style scarf. This eight-hour treatment will restore hair to pre-holiday condition.

WIND WARNING

In summer a combination of strong winds on a sandy beach can cause as much damage as the sun, so occasionally use a good "leave-in conditioner" on your hair for the day. Choose one that contains Vitamin B5, which will nourish and protect your hair from beach damage.

Beauty on a Budget

LEARN TO LOOK GORGEOUS FOR LESS with these money-saving tips for all your beauty needs. Including thrifty tips and tactics for skin, hair, make-up and bodycare, as well as the products that are worth spending money on and the ones that aren't, this chapter will help you be frugal without forfeiting good looks and glamour. .

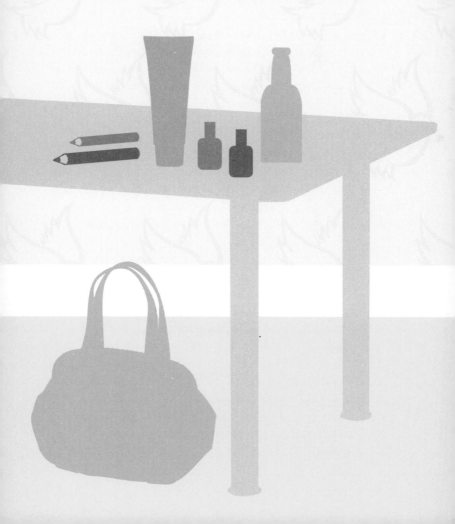

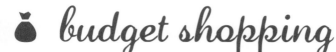 **budget shopping**

DISCOVER WHAT'S IMPORTANT TO YOU

Make two lists – one detailing the products you really can't live without and one of the items that you don't use very much or really don't need to use. For example, if you have dry skin you'll need a good moisturizer but can quite happily go without toner. Or if you hate your pale lashes, you'll need mascara but perhaps wouldn't miss lipliner. You may end up halving your beauty bill.

LOYALTY IS NOT ALWAYS A VIRTUE

Just because you can't live without your favourite expensive moisturizer, it doesn't necessarily mean you have to buy all your skincare products from the same range. Rather than being fiercely loyal to one brand, experiment with supermarket own-brand products for basic beauty items such as deodorant, toner and eye make-up remover.

PRIORITIZE THE PROBLEM

Is your hair dry or greasy? If it's dry it might be worth buying a budget shampoo and spending a bit more on conditioner. However, if your hair is greasy it makes more sense to go for a shampoo that targets your problem and to save money on a budget conditioner.

NEED NOT WANT

Learn to prioritize. Yes, that metallic eyeliner is tempting but it's not going to make you look any prettier if you haven't got a good canvas on which to apply it. When money is tight, make sure you have the basics to keep you groomed and glowing before splashing out on sparkly extras.

SOMETIMES IT PAYS...

Many department stores and supermarkets offer reward cards on which you collect points for every purchase you make. Collect points while buying essentials like soap and toothpaste and when you've collected enough you can use them to get a free beauty treat.

BULK-BUY

Take advantage of promotions. Stock up on six months' worth
of shampoo and conditioner the next time your favourite line of
products is on offer at a reduced price. However, some products –
mascara, for example – have a short shelf life so don't buy them in
bulk or they'll go to waste.

CUT BACK ON NEUTRALS

It's worth splashing out on expensive brands when buying brighter eye
and lip shades as cheaper make-up sinks into your skin more, making
the colour less vibrant on application. But when buying neutral colours,
don't splash the cash – you'll get the same effect from cheaper ranges.

SIGN UP FOR SAVINGS

Many make-up brands offer regular benefits, such as free full-size
samples, to people on their mailing lists. If you don't want spam
clogging up your inbox, open a new email account specifically for
mailing lists – and log on whenever you're in need of a freebie!

SUPERSIZE SHAMPOO

When buying shampoo or face wash, you may save money in the
short term by buying smaller bottles, but it's often wiser to go for the
biggest available size if it's a product you already know and trust. Try
working out the cost wash for wash to discover how much you'll save.

KEEP IT SIMPLE

Trying every product in the quest for a perfect complexion may be
tempting, but overdoing the experimental purchases is one of the
biggest – and priciest – beauty mistakes. Keep it simple with a good and
trusted cleanser, moisturizer and sunscreen – the rest is unnecessary.

PARE DOWN

There's an alarming array of mascaras out there – ones that lengthen,
volumize, curl or separate. Don't be tempted to buy one of each. You'll
only use one at a time. Also, once opened mascaras must be used
within three months, so having unused options is simply wasteful.

DON'T GET KITTED OUT

Make-up brands are always trying to create complete product packages that look like a bargain, but don't get sucked in. Chances are you'll only end up using two or three things from the kit, and you could have saved money and got more of the things you really liked by buying them individually.

COMPARE THE MARKET

If you have seen the perfect shade of eyeshadow or lipstick at an expensive make-up counter, ask for a sample and then compare it to cheaper brands. Chances are you'll find exactly the same colour for a fraction of the price.

SAVE ON SHAMPOO

It's essentially just soap, so expensive miracle formulas are unlikely to give you noticeably better results than a basic version. Most supermarkets and chemists do their own-branded ranges these days with products targeted specifically for different hair

BUY COLOUR IN BULK

If you know you want to achieve a certain look – say smoky eyes – it can actually be cheaper to buy an eyeshadow palette that contains all the shades you'll need to create the look rather than individual colours.

CHEAPER FOUNDATION

You don't need an exact colour match for tinted moisturizers, or even much in the way of coverage, so save your money and buy a cheaper high street version for results that are just as good.

COMPARE INGREDIENTS

You love your expensive moisturizer because it leaves your skin super-smooth, but are you sure you're paying for a quality product and not just for packaging and the name? Compare the ingredients with cheaper brands and you're sure to find a cheaper product that works just as well.

GET GLOSSY FOR LESS

You're either going to lick lip gloss off, or leave it behind on coffee cups or people's cheeks, whether it's expensive or cheap. Save your pennies and buy a budget one!

SMOOTH MOVE

There's no point splashing out on an expensive body moisturizer, as you want to be able to slather it on daily without worrying about how much you are using. Inexpensive body lotions and oils will do just as much to moisturize your skin as the cheaper brands – but they just might not smell as expensive!

DON'T GET SUCKERED

Special offers such as 'two-for-one' are only bargains if you're actually going to use the products. If you're just going to put them in the back of a drawer and forget about them, that's not saving!

BE BRAND SAVVY

If you are looking for a particular brand of make-up, don't just buy it from the first place you see it. Different stores sell the same products at different prices, so shop around. And don't forget the Internet – specialist beauty-product websites and eBay offer massive savings.

DON'T BE A MAGPIE

Are you a sucker for pretty packaging? Well, the truth is cheap doesn't have to mean ugly. You can keep your bathroom looking beautiful by transferring cheap products into pretty bottles.

NAIL IT DOWN

The more expensive nail varnishes often contain stronger colour pigments so you can apply fewer coats and the colour won't chip as quickly, which means a small bottle will go a long way. They are also more likely to glide on smoothly for a better finish.

A NATURAL BLUSH

In bronzers and blushers, the powder tends to be of a finer grade in more expensive brands, so the colour will look more natural on your cheeks and should last longer. Cheaper brands are more likely to clump and streak.

CONCEAL THE TRUTH

Cheaper brands of concealer tend to dry out quickly, which can make the blemish you were trying to conceal stand out even more, or accentuate those undereye bags.

SPEND ON SELF-TANNERS

It's worth spending a little more on self-tanners to avoid the nasty smell of cheaper brands and ensure a streak-free finish – you'll still be spending less than if you had it applied professionally.

ANY KIND WILL DO

Cosmetic powder doesn't have to be expensive – the translucent version of any budget brand will do the trick. Luxury brands may be ground finer and available in various shades, but a translucent variety covers most people's needs.

KEEP KOHL

Even expensive eyeliner can smudge, and the ingredients in the cheaper versions are almost identical if you compare them.

SPEND FOR YOUR AGE

Younger skins can get away with cheaper foundation, but if you're hoping to hide wrinkles and age spots it's worth paying more as the higher-end formulations tend to be more hydrating and contain the latest light-reflecting technology.

TREAT YOUR FACE

A good day facial moisturizer will leave your face smooth and therefore cut down on the amount of foundation you need as well as any primer products you may have to buy.

basic beauty tools

BEAUTY IN A BOX

Store all your make-up in an airtight container to seal out moisture, which can change the appearance and texture of some make-up. Excess moisture can even lead to make-up going off, meaning you will have to throw it away and replace it.

BALLS IN A BAG

We tend to throw away make-up bags when they inevitably get grubby but you can ensure your make-up bag lasts longer simply by putting two or three cotton balls in it. The cotton balls attract all of the loose powder or lipstick in your bag, keeping it cleaner for longer.

CLEVER COTTON

Cotton buds (swabs) are inexpensive but invaluable as they make a very versatile make-up tool. They are great for applying eyeshadow, blending in foundation and concealer and for fixing eyeliner and mascara mistakes; you can also use them for touching up manicures.

WASH AND BRUSH UP

The key to long-lasting make-up brushes that don't need constant replacing is regular cleaning. Soak your brushes in hot water with a mild liquid soap, then rinse under cold running water. Leave out on a paper towel to air-dry. Snip away frayed ends to ensure flawless application.

PAINT-STORE PARADISE

If you go to an art supply store you'll be able to find brushes in the same shapes and sizes as make-up brushes but for half the price. Be careful though – not all paintbrushes are suitable for use on your face so make sure you pick brushes with soft bristles and choose natural fibres rather than synthetics.

beauty gadgets: not worth your cash

BODY-TONING PADS

If you want to lose weight these gadgets just won't help. Even if their mild toning effect does anything in the way of tightening, because fat sits on top of muscle you won't see any difference unless you diet and exercise too.

HOME-TANNING SYSTEMS

You can achieve just as good results with the latest spray-tan product bought from a pharmacy (aerosol sprays are best on hard-to-reach areas) as you can with expensive home-tanning systems.

MASSAGE GADGETS

When it comes to massages, nothing beats the human touch. Skin-on-skin contact adds to the relaxation factor and you can achieve a greater range of pressure and strokes with your hands than with any fancy, costly gadgets.

ELECTRIC MANICURE SET

Electric nail files are pricey and can actually split your nails. It's much easier and cheaper to do it manually, with the ever-reliable emery board under your own steam.

HEATED EYELASH CURLERS

Just blast your normal eyelash curlers under your hairdryer for a second instead. But to avoid singed eyelashes make sure the curlers are not too hot before using them.

FACIAL SAUNA

You can achieve exactly the same results with a bowl of warm water and a towel over your head. Add a few drops of essential oil to the water and you can create your own soothing facial sauna for a fraction of the price.

HOT STYLE

Blow drying wet hair and then styling it can cause damage and lead to breakages. It's much better to let your hair dry naturally before using heated stylers.

FEET TREATS

Foot spas are waste of cash with weakly powered bubbles! Simply fill a plastic bowl with enough warm water to cover your feet and add some softening bubble bath for an equivalent experience.

ILLUMINATED COSMETIC MIRROR

Beauty mirrors can be expensive and bulbs need replacing. It's much better to apply make-up in natural light anyway, or you can risk looking like a clown when you leave the house. To get an even better effect than an illuminated cosmetic mirror, simply position your mirror next to a window and place a lamp nearby.

INDUSTRIAL-STRENGTH HAIRDRYER

Hairstylists use expensive super-strength hairdryers with powerful motors because they blow-dry so many clients every day, but you don't need that much power to achieve the same finish at home, and these types can damage hair if used regularly.

beauty gadgets:
worth every penny

HAIRSTYLING SCISSORS
You can't use any old scissors to trim your fringe (bangs). Cutting fabric
and paper blunts the blades so they'll snag and split your hair. A pair of
professional-quality blades will save you a fortune in salon trims.

MAGNIFYING MIRRORS
They make everything – from plucking your eyebrows to applying
your make-up – so much easier. So investing in a good magnifying
mirror will make it simple to take care of your beauty at home.

ELECTRIC TOOTHBRUSH
Nothing says 'well groomed' better than a pearly white smile. An
electric toothbrush shifts much more bacteria than brushing with a
regular brush, saving you a small fortune in dentist bills.

PEDOMETER
Clipped onto your belt this gadget will count the amount of steps you
do a day. Think of it as your own motivational personal trainer – but
much cheaper! Aim to do 10,000 steps a day to stay in shape.

BIKINI TRIMMER
Specifically designed for use on sensitive skin, this gadget allows
you to trim and shape with precision. Investing in one of these nifty
gadgets will save you a fortune each month on salon bikini waxes.

HAIRDRYER WITH SETTINGS

Having different heat settings will set your style and protect your hair from excessive heat exposure. Look out for hairdryers with ionic conditioning to help reduce frizz and static. Just think how much money you'll save on salon blow-dries.

HAIR-REMOVAL SYSTEMS

These home systems are perfect for small areas of the body. Needle-free, they use gentle laser or pulsed light and although they're not cheap to buy, in comparison to having regular electrolysis at a salon you'll save a fortune.

CERAMIC STRAIGHTENERS

Worth the money, ceramic straighteners protect hair from static and snagging. Plus, they heat up quickly, removing the need to go over the same section of hair numerous times, and therefore are gentler on your hair. Also, by wrapping your hair around the straightening iron you can create bouncy curls. Two tools for the price of one!

EXERCISE DVDS

If you want a cheap aerobic workout, exercise DVDs are great. You'll be able to afford a huge variety for less than one month's gym membership and class fees. Or make it even cheaper and sign up to a DVD rental website.

DECENT TWEEZERS

A good-quality pair of tweezers will last you forever. You'll be able to shape perfectly arched eyebrows without the help of a professional, so these inexpensive tools will pay for themselves in no time.

active ingredients: worth every penny

CERAMIDES
A natural substance within the skin, ceramides reduce natural water loss of the skin by forming a protective barrier, and also help to hold the skin's cells together in a firm, smooth structure. Ceramides can also be produced synthetically and added to skincare products, and have been used in products since the early 1990s. They have proven anti-ageing benefits.

RETINOIDS
These vitamin-A derivatives are one of the few ingredients shown to combat the serious signs of ageing. They penetrate skin more deeply, to strengthen and replenish collagen and elastin, plump up skin and unclog pores.

DIHYDROXYACETONE
Present in self-tanners, this carbohydrate reacts with amino acids found in the top layers of the skin to create a shade of brown within two to six hours, and can build colour depth with every reapplication. It has a long history of safe use. A cost-effective and healthy way to tan.

ALPHA-LIPOIC ACID
A powerful antioxidant and anti-inflammatory that occurs naturally in your cells and helps reduce under-eye puffiness. An excellent ingredient to look out for in eye creams.

VITAMIN E

This nutrient plays a crucial role in protecting skin cells from environmental damage on an everyday basis, but it is also excellent for calming stressed, sun-damaged skin.

ALPHA-HYDROXY ACIDS (AHAS)

AHAs, originally derived from fruits, reduce fine lines, smooth skin and remove blemishes. They also help exfoliate without the need for scrubbing. AHAs need time to work – go for products that you leave on the skin, such as moisturizers and masks. They can be harsh though, so avoid them if you have sensitive skin.

ZINC OXIDE

Zinc oxide is a proven UV blocker. It's the basis of many sunscreens and is particularly good if you have sensitive skin.

BETA HYDROXY ACID (BHA OR SALICYLIC ACID)

Found naturally in plants, this is a great ingredient for blemish-prone skin. It has antibacterial properties and gently exfoliates deep inside your pores to prevent outbreaks.

CAFFEINE

Caffeine helps ingredients penetrate the skin and can stimulate the circulation. It's most widely used in cellulite treatments, but is also useful in gels to combat puffy eyes.

VITAMIN B3

Also known as niacin, B3 has been shown to prevent skin from losing water, keeping it hydrated. Worth paying for.

ingredients that are a waste of money

HUMECTANTS

These moisturizing additives are actually more important in preventing your product from drying out than for keeping your skin moisturized!

ENZYMES

Used in skincare for exfoliation and to inhibit free-radical damage. However, enzymes are picky about what conditions they will work in and often need other enzymes, called coenzymes, to function, or a specific temperature or pH. Unlikely to do much, so save your cash.

OXYGEN

Oxygen boosts skin cell turnover when you breathe it in, not when you apply it to your skin. Steer clear!

ALL NATURAL

When a product claims that it contains only natural ingredients, it's not saying that the contents are safer for your skin. All it really means is that the ingredients were not produced chemically. However, this doesn't mean that it will be better for your skin or never cause allergic reactions.

PEPTIDES

These flash-sounding ingredients haven't been proven to fight ageing, so it's not worth paying more for them.

POLYPHENOLS

Again, these are great antioxidants with anti-inflammatory benefits when consumed in things such as green tea, but they've not yet been shown to offer the same benefit when slathered on your skin.

DNA

Including the building blocks of all life in a skincare product is pointless because as an ingredient it can't affect a cell at a genetic level – and nor would you want it to!

OMEGAS-3 AND -6

Essential fatty acids such as omega-3 and 6 give you glowing skin when eaten in oily fish and nuts, but they haven't been shown to have a significant effect when applied to your skin's surface.

make-up makeover

END OF LINES

Ask your local beauty salon for end-of-line lipsticks and nail polishes. They'll often offer them at a discount to clear the shelves for new stock.

DITCH THE FANCY PRODUCTS

Let's face it, tried-and-tested products may not be fashionable but they've been around for years, they don't break the bank and they work. And that's why they've been around for years.

COUNT ON COUNTERS

Department store make-up counters are always happy to offer free makeovers so why not make the most of them by booking one just before a special occasion? Don't feel you have to buy anything, but you will sometimes get a discount on any purchases that you make.

COLOUR ME CUT-PRICE

Makeover salons that help you decide on colours for clothes and make-up are often much quieter in the late summer months and early winter (Christmas, New Year and spring tend to be busiest). Look for special offers or simply drive a hard bargain and demand a discount – starting at half price.

THROW A MAKE-UP PARTY

Companies selling make-up door-to-door will often organize make-up parties and come to your home if you can guarantee a certain number of guests. So invite the girls, open a bottle of wine and make it an evening. Anything you buy will be discounted.

COLOUR-MATCH YOURSELF

If you can't afford to visit a special salon to be told which colours suit you, buy a book of colour swatches. By holding the colours up against your face you get a great idea of which shades of eye make-up, lipstick and blusher to experiment with.

MAKEOVER MATES

We all have make-up mistakes, freebies from magazines and unwanted presents lurking somewhere, but don't throw something away just because the colour doesn't suit you – it might be perfect for a friend. Have a product swap party and invite friends to bring their make-up mistakes along. When inviting them make it clear that the make-up must be new and unsealed. Sharing make-up or using old make-up that may have deteriorated can be a health hazard.

DON'T ASK, DON'T GET

When splashing out your cash on a new exfoliator, see if the girls behind the make-up counter will throw in a complimentary moisturizer for you to use afterwards. They can only say no!

BE A GUINEA PIG

Offer yourself as a test dummy at your local beauty college. Trainee make-up artists can practise creating a look on you for free. Chances are you'll look fabulous, but don't worry if it all goes horribly wrong – it will easily wash off!

WRITE A LETTER

It's always worth writing in to newspapers and magazines for a reader makeover. They often have to find at least one real-life case study for every issue and so welcome volunteers. You'll be pampered and preened (and photographed!) for free.

UNEARTH YOUR ANTIQUES

Every woman's got one – a huge drawer that holds lots of unused make-up. Now's a great time to tip it all out. You'll be amazed by how much you own; how much is usable; and how much you actually like. Mascara and eyeliner should only be kept three to six months, so these need to go if older than this.

MAKE YOUR OWN WAVES

No need to have a perm in a salon to get a curly new look. Instead, do it at home by splitting hair into sections and wrapping each section around a rag. Pin up until dry or leave overnight and you will wake up to beautiful, tousled tresses.

ONLINE MAKEOVER

A whole host of beauty websites now offer a free online tool (often called a Virtual Makeover) that lets you see how you would look with different hairstyles, lipstick colours, sunglasses, hats etc. You simply scan in a picture of yourself and experiment to your heart's content. It's free and fun.

CHANGE ONE THING

People assume you need to change your whole make-up bag for a new look, but just tweaking one small thing can have an amazing effect – and save you money. Investing in one new staple, such as a green eyeliner or a different shade of lipstick, will refresh your other products.

SAVVY SAMPLES

It's important to see foundation in natural light to ensure you've chosen the right shade. Ask for samples at beauty counters to give a new colour a trial run. This will avoid a costly mistake and you may well end up with enough for a few nights out!

BENEFITS OF A RESTYLE

If you can't afford to splash out on a full cut, a cheap and effective way to restyle is to have your fringe (bangs) cut. A fringe is nearly always in fashion and can really change your look, plus hairstylists charge a fraction of the price of a whole haircut to create one.

multipurpose products

LINE THEM UP
Want a smoky-eyed look without buying a new eyeliner? With your eye closed, touch the tip of a mascara wand along the lash line of your upper eyelid, then quickly smudge the dots with a cotton bud (swab) for smoky definition.

THRIFTY THREE-IN-ONES
NARS invented the original multipurpose colour stick, which can be used on lips, cheeks and eyes. Now other ranges, including supermarket own brands, have jumped on the three-in-one band-wagon, so you can get this make-up must-have for a fraction of the cost.

SUPER-STRAIGHT
Forget lots of fancy hair tools – you can achieve a multitude of styles with just a thin straightening iron. As well as poker-straight locks you can create corkscrew curls by wrapping your hair around one plate of the iron, working your way up towards the roots. You can also vary the look depending on how tightly you wind your hair or by brushing out the curls to create soft waves.

HANDY HIGHLIGHTERS
Highlighters are a great budget buy as they can be used in so many ways. To lift your eyes – apply along the brow bone; for a wide-eyed look – apply to the inner corner of your eyes; for a healthy glow – blend along your cheekbones; and for full lips – blend along your Cupid's bow.

SUPER STAINS
Many make-up brands now offer multipurpose stains that can be applied to both the cheeks and lips. This saves the cost of buying two products and creates a more natural rosy glow.

EXOTIC EYELINER

Eyeshadow is available in a far wider selection of colours than eyeliner. Be creative and save money by turning your favourite shade of eyeshadow into an eyeliner. Simply dampen an eyeliner brush with water, dip it into the shadow and run along your lashes.

PERFECT HIDEAWAY

Don't despair if you've run out of concealer, try the ring of foundation that collects around the neck of your foundation bottle. Moisture that was in the foundation will have evaporated, so the remnants are more concentrated and will offer better coverage – just like concealer.

MAGIC ANTI-STATIC SPRAY

Hairspray can be used to tame unruly clothes as well as unruly hair. The aerosol spray can prevent static build-up, so when wearing a silky dress simply spritz a bit of hairspray on to your tights (pantyhose).

REPURPOSE PRODUCTS

If you run out of essential items some products can double up – bronzer can be used as blusher or eyeshadow and mild shampoo as a make-up brush cleaner.

MULTIPURPOSE MASCARA

Get more out of your mascara by using it to groom and define eyebrows as well as lashes. Go for a clear mascara or pick a natural-looking colour, as black may be too harsh for some complexions.

LUSCIOUS LIPS

Don't want to waste money on yet another lipstick? Cream or powder blusher can be dabbed on lips with a finger to create a soft, sensual look. For a creamier texture, top the blusher with clear gloss or petroleum jelly.

LIPPY CHEEKS

Lipstick can also be used as a blusher – but bear in mind that lipstick contains far more pigment than blusher. To avoid going overboard, start with a tiny dab, then gradually build up the colour. Blend well with your fingertips or a cotton bud.

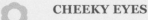

CHEEKY EYES

Warm tones really open up the eye area. So instead of buying a new eyeshadow, apply powder blusher in a soft bronze, peach or rose colour to your eyelids up to your brow bone. Using the same colour on your eyes and cheeks will even out your skin tone and give you a natural-looking glow.

A DYNAMIC DUO

For the ultimate budget-friendly look, make up your whole face using only bronzing powder and petroleum jelly. Use the bronzer as blusher and eyeshadow, then mix it with some petroleum jelly for a golden lip gloss. Finally, slick some petroleum jelly on your lashes and brows for shine and definition.

NOT JUST FOR BABIES

There's a host of overpriced fancy body oils and sprays on the market, but all you really need is a little baby oil. Rub it in after a shower or add a few drops to your bath water for super-soft skin. It also works as cuticle cream.

WISE WIPES

Keep on hand a packet of three-in-one face wipes that cleanse, tone and moisturize, or at least cleanse and tone. By choosing a multipurpose product rather than three separate ones you'll save money and time.

HANDY FRIZZ FIGHTER

Hand lotion doesn't just soothe dry mitts, it can also smooth dry hair. Apply the lotion to hands as normal and then simply run your hands over the frizzy area. The moisturizers in the lotion will instantly smooth out frizz, leaving behind a glossy sheen.

WELL POLISHED

Always keep a bottle of clear nail polish in your handbag (purse). Not only does it add smart gloss to nails in seconds when you've no time for colour, it will also stop runs in tights (panty hose) from getting worse if you dab a little on to the ends of the run.

A POINTED RESPONSE

Invest in a medium-sized brush with a slanted tip for the ultimate multiple-use tool. You can use the angled edge for eyeshadow and the fatter side for blusher and loose power. Do be sure to clean your brushes regularly and between different uses.

bases & concealers

CLEVER COMBO

Why pay for a separate foundation and moisturizer, when you can get one product that does both jobs: a tinted moisturizer? To ensure a natural look, test it down the centre of your nose to make sure it settles well around your pores.

LIQUID GOLD

To get to the last bit of liquid concealer in a tube with a wand applicator, use a concealer brush or a clean lip brush.

SHADES OF SUMMER

Instead of buying a new foundation in the summer months when your skin is a darker shade, mix your old one with a little bronzer and moisturizer in the palm of your hand and apply to give skin a healthy glow.

FINGERTIP FOUNDATION

There's no need to splash out on special sponges for foundation application. With practice you can achieve a flawless finish using only your fingers. Fingers can reach places that sponges can't and it's also easier to avoid getting foundation in your eyebrows and hairline.

COLOUR CODED

A cheap foundation will work just as well as an expensive one if you choose the right shade. Don't bother testing it on the back of your hand – the skin colour is too different. Instead, pop a blob onto your jawline. Provided it blends seamlessly into your neck, it's the right choice regardless of price.

FATTEN UP YOUR FOUNDATION

To make your foundation last longer, mix a small amount with your daily moisturizer before applying. You'll achieve the perfect tint of colour that spreads on easily to even out your complexion.

THE UNDERTONES

Rather than slapping on lots of beige concealer, go for a small dab of a shade with an undertone that will neutralize your blemish or dark circles, and will last a lot longer. A green undertone counteracts redness, yellow conceals dark circles and lilac lifts sallow skin.

GET TO THE BOTTOM OF THINGS

If you can't get to that last bit of foundation or squeeze the last liquid make-up out of the tube, place it under hot running water for a few seconds. The warmth should help it slide out.

LIGHTEN UP

We all love YSL's Touche Éclat for hiding our dark under-eye circles but it's not cheap. Check out other ranges, including supermarket own-brand cosmetics, as nearly all of them do an imitation. Not as expensively packaged perhaps, but many are just as effective.

DON'T HIGHLIGHT PROBLEMS

Again, there's a myth that foundation needs to go all over the face. It doesn't. Foundation can be spot-applied to the areas where you need to even out your skin tone, such as grey under-eye bags or blotchy cheeks. This gives a more natural look to your make-up and means you use less.

STICK TO IT

Get the last bit of concealer stick out of the bottom of the tube with a toothpick – but make sure you apply it to your hand first. Don't use the toothpick on your face!

BACK TO LIFE

Has your foundation become caked and dry? Pour a few drops of alcohol-free toner into your foundation bottle and shake. It will last that bit longer and you'll be toning your face at the same time.

DITCH THE EXTRAS

Some cosmetic companies charge as much for a face primer as for their foundation – promising that it will ensure a smooth application and long-lasting finish. Don't be fooled – your normal moisturizer will do exactly the same job.

BLEMISH SOLUTION

If you suffer from oily skin and blemishes, think twice before buying overpriced medicated foundations. Stick to the one you love and simply add a few drops of witch hazel. Known for its astringent properties and for tightening pores, it's often used in toners for oily skin and is available in pharmacies.

BE SIZE SAVVY

When you shop for foundations and concealers, don't just compare the prices. Write down how many millilitres/ounces they give you and figure out the cost per millilitre/ounce to accurately compare prices. If you don't do this the prices – and bottle sizes – can be deceiving.

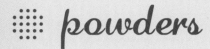 # powders

SKIP A STAGE
If you have dry or mature skin don't bother with face powder.
Foundation doesn't need 'setting' these days to stay put and powder
can settle in creases and dry areas to give an unflattering effect.

DOUBLE-DUTY BEAUTY
The latest mineral powders are made from natural ingredients, are
gentle on skin, and replace the need for foundation as they offer great
matt coverage. Perfect for oilier skins.

TREATMENT MAKE-UP
Buy powder that contains an SPF and moisturizing ingredients so you
get more bang for your buck.

MAKE USE OF LEFTOVERS
Once you've finished your loose or pressed powder, the sponge applicator
makes a great oil blotter for greasy hair roots between washes.

PUT A CAP ON IT
Some make-up companies recommend buying loose power to keep at
home and a pressed powder compact to keep in your handbag (purse).
Save money by just buying the far more versatile loose variety and a
retractable brush that can hold a little powder in the cap.

POWDER RUN DRY?

Loose powder tends to be more expensive than pressed powder but if you don't wear much, you can make your own. Mix baby powder with one part powder from a cheap powder compact. Choose the compact powder in a colour darker than your skin and mix to get the right shade.

BE A PEARLY QUEEN

To make a 'luminescent' face powder for evenings, add a little white or peach frosted eyeshadow to a small amount of face powder in your palm and apply with a brush. If you prefer, you can just dust your face very lightly with any of these frosted powders using a brush.

MAGIC POWDER

Run out of foundation? Make a substitute of two parts face powder to one part unscented hand lotion. Mix only enough for a single use in the palm of your hand. It has a nice finish, but the oil in the lotion can darken the colour, so you may need to add some baby powder to lighten it.

ADD SOME DEPTH

If you have old loose power that's a shade too light so it's not getting used, add some bronzer or blusher to it. Just add a little at a time and mix to create a bespoke colour that is perfect for your skin tone.

CLEVER CONTAINERS

Wash out pretty powder pots once they're empty and use them to store earrings or cotton balls.

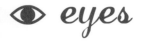 # eyes

TAPE FOR PERFECTION
Low-tack masking tape can safely create the perfect lines for precise liquid eyeliner. The trick is to cut a piece about 2.5 cm (1 in) long and peel it off the skin of your hand once or twice to lose a little of the stickiness. Then place at the desired angle on the corners of your eyes.

GOOD FOUNDATIONS
You don't need to spend extortionate amounts on expensive bases and primers that promise to stop your eyeshadow creasing and flaking. Simply apply your foundation to your eyelid as a base to keep your shadow in place all day.

GO FOR GOLD
Gold shimmer eyeshadow can be used as a highlight all over the face. Run it along the bony bit just below the eyebrow or dab it down the centre line of the nose and at the top of the cheekbones. But try to stick to only two areas of shine at a time!

REFRESH MASCARA
You can refresh dried-out mascara by heating with a hairdryer for a few seconds. However, make sure you change your mascara every three to six months to avoid nasty eye infections.

MAKE WAVES WITHOUT CURLERS
You don't need expensive eyelash curlers to curl your lashes. Just bend your lashes back from the root with your finger, and hold them there for a few seconds. Set the curl with a coat of mascara.

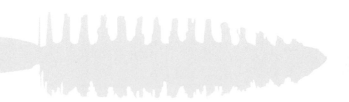

SHADOW FIXES

Keep your eyeliner in place, and reduce the need for constant reapplication, by patting dabs of black eyeshadow on top of it. This will stop your eyeliner smudging or bleeding and will make your precious kohl stick last that bit longer.

WIPE AWAY MISTAKES

Forget expensive eye make-up removing wipes, which can often sting and irritate the face. Low-cost baby wipes, which are often used by make-up artists, work just as well and are often a lot gentler.

AFTERNOON CLEAN-UP

A cotton bud (swab) dipped in petroleum jelly or lip balm is a great way to clean up smudged eye make-up, thereby avoiding that bad mid-afternoon habit of washing everything off and reapplying – a sure-fire way to use up products twice as fast. Make sure you don't get any in your eyes!

REFRIGERATOR FRESH

Try keeping eye pencils, lipsticks and nail polishes in the refrigerator. This will stop them drying out and make them easier to apply. It should also prevent the tips of pencils and lipsticks from breaking off.

EYE DYE DO-IT-YOURSELF

Instead of going to a beautician, tint your eyelashes and eyebrows with a home kit that is far cheaper than a trip to a salon.

BUDGET MASCARA

Of all the make-up products, mascara is the one you can scrimp on because the secret to good mascara is the brush not the formula. Many cheaper brands have very good mascaras.

DON'T LASH OUT

Fond of false lashes? Be economical and get a better effect by snipping the lashes in half and placing them only on the outside of the eye. Don't place them at the very end of the lash line, though, or your falsies are liable to droop – leave a 2 mm ($^1/_{16}$ in) gap instead.

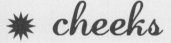 cheeks

TOTAL TAN

Wear a bronzer all year round. We tend to think of it as a summertime treat but it's a Hollywood secret that keeps many an ageing starlet from looking her age. And the subtle, healthy glow will save you lots of money on tanning treatments.

FIRST FLUSH

Don't overdo it with the blusher – you only need to use a tiny amount provided you apply it correctly. The area to apply it to is the 'apples' of your cheeks, where you blush, funnily enough!

TONE IT DOWN

Powder blusher too bright? Don't throw it out. Crush it up and mix in a little brown blusher, matt brown eyeshadow or matt powdered bronzer.

LIGHTEN UP

Powder blusher too dark? You can lighten it a couple of shades by crushing it up and mixing in a little baby or face powder.

HAVE A REFILL

Many make-up companies now make eco-friendly, reusable compacts with refills that can cost a lot less than buying a new compact every time.

FIND YOUR PERFECT PARTNER

Don't waste money on lots of different shades of blusher – if you find the right shade to complement your skin tone you can wear it day and night. Fair-skinned ladies should go for pink and tawny tones, redheads will glow in peach and coral shades, and olive skin tones suit brown and copper shades.

DO A REPAIR JOB

Eyeshadow, blusher or powder that comes inside a compact may start to break up and fall out in time. This can be fixed by adding a little surgical spirit (rubbing alcohol) and smoothing the powder back in place with a butter knife. Let the powder dry completely before using.

lips

GET LIPPY

There's no need to pay extra for long-lasting lipstick. Even the cheapest lipstick can last all night if you apply it well. Use a lip pencil all over the lips, then apply face powder to set the pencil. Top with a coat of lipstick, then blot your lips by pressing them together on some tissue before applying a second coat.

DON'T BE FLAKY

Instead of splashing cash on a lip primer, use a touch of petroleum jelly before applying lipstick. Dip an old toothbrush in petroleum jelly and gently rub it over your lips in a circular motion to scrub away all the flaky bits.

TEA TONER

Tea can help your lips retain moisture and appear smoother. Simply press a used teabag to clean lips, while it's still warm, and use to clean for five minutes.

LINE BY LINE

A lipliner can be used in the place of lipstick to colour in the entire lip. As well as taking up less space in your handbag (purse), the colour lasts longer.

LONG-LIFE LIPSTICK

Lipstick can last for up to two years, depending on the brand, so don't throw it out when you only have a little nub left. Scrape it into an empty, sterilized lip-gloss or eyeshadow pot instead. If you're feeling creative, you could even mix different shades to make your own colour. Apply with a lipbrush.

BROWN SUGAR

If your lips are dry, a budget, soothing balm can be made by mixing a little brown sugar with honey. The sugar will gently exfoliate dead skin cells while the honey is great for rehydrating dry skin.

MIX IT UP

You can make your own lip gloss from the end of a lipstick. Put a little petroleum jelly and a little of your leftover lipstick in an empty, sterilized lip-gloss pot. If it doesn't blend together well, put it in a microwave-safe container and heat for a few seconds.

KEEP IT CLEAN

When applying a clear gloss over coloured lipstick, always apply using a cotton bud (swab), not the applicator in the gloss tube. Dip the cotton bud (swab) just once into the gloss and then apply to your lips. This prevents the rest of your gloss becoming discoloured and you having to throw it away before it's finished.

SPICY LIP PLUMPER

Cinnamon encourages blood flow, and is the key ingredient in many expensive lip plumpers. Blend a drop of cinnamon oil with a tablespoon of olive or almond oil and rub it onto your lips. It will make your lips tingle and give them a natural fullness.

BETTER BRUSH STROKES

Use a lip brush to apply your lipstick. With a lip brush, you will apply a thinner layer of lipstick than if you were to apply it straight out of the tube. Plus you can scrape out every last bit of your lipstick with your lip brush, preventing leftovers. Waste not, want not.

THE PERFECT SHADE

Have a too-bright lipstick you'd like to salvage? Apply a medium-brown lipstick or lipliner pencil over the top to tone it down.

NATURAL OILS

A little olive oil will soothe dry, chapped lips as well as any store-bought balm. Simply dab it on with your finger.

GO GREEN

If you recycle your old lipstick tubes some companies, such as MAC, will give you a new lipstick for free (if you return six empties).

CAP IT

Taking care of your lipsticks will make them last longer. To avoid squashing it, make sure your lipstick is rolled all the way down before putting the cap on. Also, make sure the top clicks into place to keep out air and reduce the growth of bacteria.

SHIMMER AND SHINE

Make your own sparkly lip gloss: stir 1 heaped teaspoon of petroleum jelly, ¼ teaspoon of hot, boiled water and 1 teaspoon of sugar together until the sugar is dissolved. Then add some pink or red food colouring and a pinch of edible glitter. Let the mixture cool then scoop it into an empty lip-gloss container. Use within one month.

LIP SERVICE

If a broken lipstick is too mangled or misshapen to go back in the tube smoothly, use a small knife to transfer the lipstick to a plastic art palette. You can pick up artists' palettes at your local art store for next to nothing.

cleansing & care

CLEVER CLEANSING

If you cleanse your skin properly you'll save a load of money on blemish
treatments and super-creams. Always wash your hands first – dirty
palms make for clogged pores. Be especially gentle around your eyes, as
dragging on this skin will lead to wrinkles and ageing crow's feet.

GET CLARIFICATION

'Clarifying' mists and lotions often contain harsh ingredients such
as acids and alcohol, which could make your skin feel sore and look
blotchy. Cheaper products that don't make these claims may actually
be better for your skin. Check the ingredients and make sure they're
alcohol-free.

TONE UP

Most store-bought soaps are alkaline relative to the skin. A dirt-cheap
way to redress this balance is by using diluted vinegar as a toner.

KITCHEN CLEANSER

Why buy an expensive cleanser when you can make one at home
that's suitable for all skin types? This simple mixture will cleanse,
tone and smooth: mix 1 teaspoon of honey with 1 teaspoon of natural
(plain) yogurt. Apply to damp skin, wash gently and then rinse with
warm water.

DEEP CLEAN

Make your daily cleanser last longer and work harder by turning it into a deep cleanser. Mix a dab of it with a pinch of oatmeal, then gently massage the mixture in circular motions on to your face. Rinse with warm water and pat dry.

MILD MAKE-UP REMOVER

Common vegetable oils are great for removing non-waterproof eye make-up. Grapeseed oil is the least likely to cause irritation. Apply using soft cotton pads, then rinse thoroughly with warm water.

SOME LIKE IT COOL

If you shower or wash your face with water that is too hot it will damage the skin's natural moisture balance, so it becomes dry and in need of more moisturizer to keep it hydrated.

SPRINKLE SOME SALT

If you suffer from oily skin, then common table salt is a great way to reduce the oiliness. You can mix it with olive oil to make a cleanser or add a teaspoon to warm water to create a mild scrub.

QUALITY NOT QUANTITY

A good cleansing routine should not need to be repeated more than once a day – doubling the life of your products. Cleanse at night and simply splash lukewarm water on to your face in the morning.

MILK IT

There are plenty of expensive oil-controlling lotions available, but not many actually work. But there's a matt miracle hiding in your medicine cabinet – milk of magnesia. Pour one or two drops onto a cotton ball and lightly pat all over your face to remove any hint of sheen.

BLOOMING MARVELLOUS

Store-bought toners often contain alcohol, which can dry the skin. Save money by making your own and you'll know exactly what you're applying. Boil 250 ml (8.5 fl oz) of water and pour it over some rose petals. Leave for an hour with a lid on, then strain into a spray bottle. Lightly spritz on your face after cleansing. Store in the refrigerator for up to a month.

SAY NO TO LUXURY CLEANSERS

Rather than buying an overpriced cleanser, spend your money on quality products that actually spend time on your face, like a moisturizer. Remember, with a cleanser, you're just washing it down the sink.

PORE-TIGHTENING TOMS

Don't waste money on fancy pore-tightening treatments for blemished skin. Purée one unripe tomato and add 1 teaspoon of honey. Gently massage into your face, then rinse. The tomato acts like an astringent to tighten pores and remove excess oil, while the honey will soften the skin. Avoid using on sensitive skins.

DEWY NOT TAUT

Over-cleansing not only drains precious products, it can leave your skin feeling taut and can reduce the effectiveness of your skin as a natural barrier, leaving you vulnerable to problems that include rashes and acne. After light cleansing your skin should feel dewy rather than tight.

GIVE IT SOME FACE

Sensitive skin only needs gentle exfoliation. Rather than buying a pricy product that may upset your skin, simply exfoliate by massaging your skin with a little bit of moisturizer and a damp facecloth.

STIMULATE YOUR SKIN

Specialist brushes – including sonic brushes! – that stimulate your skin before cleansing are the latest fad, but you can replicate the effect of the bristles simply by rubbing your face with an ordinary facecloth. Wet the cloth first and gently make small circles to boost circulation.

SKIP THE TONER

We all know the 'cleanse, tone, moisturize' mantra but if your budget is tight, consider skipping the middle step. Toners can actually dilute the good effects of a moisturizer. Use a splash of cold water instead.

IN THE SPHERE

A cheap exfoliator is often as good as an expensive one – just ensure the label says it contains 'beads' or 'spheres', which means the gritty, scrubbing ingredient is perfectly round. These are kinder to your skin than the uneven, rough particles which can be abrasive and harsh.

 moisturizing

GET THE CREAM

Aqueous cream is often prescribed by doctors for people with dry-skin conditions and it's available in pharmacies at a fraction of the price of many branded moisturizers.

CLEOPATRA'S CURE

Take a leaf out of the famous Egyptian beauty's book and bathe your skin in fresh milk for a soft, supple feel. Apply it with a cotton pad using a gentle upward motion. Leave on for a few minutes then rinse off.

FORGET THE SERUM

Deep-penetrating serums target specific problems and are recommended for very dry skin, but if you are getting good results from your regular moisturizer alone don't bother splashing the extra cash.

DISCOUNT MOISTURIZER

Many believe that an expensive moisturizer is the one product to invest in, yet the role of a moisturizer is simply to hydrate and help balance the pH. Normal skin types will flourish on a simple no-frills lotion.

THREE-IN-ONE

Don't splash out on a separate serum and moisturizer; look for a formula that treats as well as hydrates. If you find a formula that also contains an SPF you've eliminated the need for three separate products in a flash.

ADD VEGETABLE OIL

One way to make your favourite moisturizer last longer is to use a small amount of natural vegetable oil as a base first. You can also mix moisturizer with a small amount of water in the palm of your hand.

LITTLE GOES A LONG WAY

Overuse of moisturizer is as bad as not using any. Too much can lead to clogged pores and blackheads. A pea-sized amount should be enough for your whole face.

HYDRATE YOUR HOUSE

Central heating is very dehydrating for your skin so in the winter months it's a good idea to place a bowl of water in every room. This puts moisture back into the atmosphere and saves you spending on extra moisturizer.

MAKE YOUR OWN OIL

Steal a trick from aromatherapy and make your own facial oil with 100 ml (3.4 fl oz) of base oil such as macadamia nut, rose hip or evening primrose. Then mix in a few drops of an essential oil such as lavender for normal skin, sandalwood for oily skin or rose for dry and mature skin.

DAY AND NIGHT CREAM

Separate moisturizers for day and night are a great marketing gimmick but you only really need one cream for your skin type. Normal to oily skin types are fine with day cream, while people with dry skin can use a richer night cream for both day and night.

CHECK THE SPF

Protection from the sun is vital to prevent premature ageing of the skin so ensure that your moisturizer has a high SPF factor. You'll also save some money as you won't have to buy an expensive facial sunscreen.

MIX YOUR OWN TINT

You can spend a fortune on tinted moisturizers that promise to produce a 'natural glow' but if you mix some leftover bronzing powder together with your last bit of sunscreen you can make summer last longer and have a protective SPF built in too.

APPLY AT THE RIGHT TIME

You will need less moisturizer and it will be much more effective if you apply it at the right time. Don't wait for your skin to feel dry, apply moisturizer immediately after you wash or shower while the skin is still damp, to seal in the moisture.

TARGET AREAS

Another way to make moisturizer last longer is to only apply it to those parts of the face that really require hydration. For most people it's the forehead and cheeks that tend to be drier, while the chin rarely needs any extra moisture.

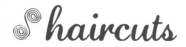 # haircuts

DO-IT-YOURSELF BLUNT FRINGE (BANGS)

Save on cost and cut your own fringe (bangs). Always cut when your hair is dry. Section off the hair you don't want to cut and tie it back. Comb your fringe down. Rest the comb on your brow bone with the teeth facing out. Don't cut your fringe any shorter than where the comb hits your face. Start 'point-cutting' – snipping at a 45-degree angle. Never cut straight across as it's impossible to keep to a perfectly straight line.

DO-IT-YOURSELF LONG FRINGE (BANGS)

Tie the rest of your hair back in a ponytail. Use a brand-new, disposable single-blade razor instead of scissors. Pull your fringe (bangs) taut between your middle and index fingers. Slide fingers all the way down to the end of your hair and then razor-cut the hair just above your fingers.

BOB IT

A style that has very little layering or is all one length, like a bob or crop, is stylish and will keep its shape as it grows, making frequent trims unnecessary. A chin-length bob will still look good when it has grown to your shoulders – which means about six months between haircuts!

SHORT OF CASH

Short, layered styles need a lot of maintenance to keep them looking good. Longer haircuts have more versatility and can be worn tied up as the style grows out. If you're going for a short chop ask your stylist for a cut that will grow out well so you don't have to return too soon.

HAIR-CUTTING CLASSES

Cutting your own hair is risky if you don't know what you're doing. Next time you visit the hair salon, ask about local hair-cutting classes or look them up on the Internet. You'll have to pay for the course, but if you stick to simple styles it could save you a fortune in hairstylist's bills in time.

LOW-COST LAYERS

Ask for a few longer layers to frame your face. This is cheaper than a completely layered style, and it should maintain its shape while growing out so you won't have to visit the salon as often.

BUDGET FOR YOUR HAIR

If you are going to spend money on just one thing to keep your hair looking beautiful, make it the haircut. A great haircut will give you a polished look, whatever products you use.

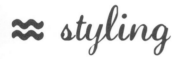

MAKE WAVES

Wavy hairstyles make it possible to put off haircuts for longer – it's harder to see grown-out layers, dark roots or split ends.

ENHANCE THE SHINE

Lavender makes a great and cheap shine-enhancing hairspray. Transfer a few drops of essential oil into a spray bottle and lightly spritz onto damp hair after washing. It will smooth the cuticles and hold your style in place – and it smells gorgeous, too.

BETTER BRUSHSTROKES

You only really need two types of brush to style your tresses: a natural-bristled round or flat brush to use on dry hair and a soft, rubber, wide-toothed comb to use on damp hair, as it stretches and snaps more easily. Brushes are inexpensive and it's worth shopping around as the right bristles will really help your hair appear smoother.

SENSIBLE BANDS

Expensive hair bands are no better for your hair than cheaper ones; just make sure they are fabric coated. Don't be tempted to use rubber bands as they can break or split hair.

BE A SWEETIE

Make your own hairspray: dissolve a tablespoon of sugar in a glass of hot water. Allow it to cool, pour the mixture into an old spray bottle and spritz evenly onto your hair to keep flyaways at bay.

GET INTO A TWIST

If your hair is naturally curly or frizzy, you can transform it into glossy ringlets at home using a little wax. While your hair is still damp, rub some wax between your fingers then take a small section of your hair and twist it around your finger. Repeat all over, for a head of fabulous curls.

ELVIS-INSPIRED

If you have short hair, a quiff is a simple, funky style that you can do yourself. Simply section a 5 cm (2 inch) portion of your hair near the front and at the top of your head. Pull the hair back and then forward in a sliding motion until you get the desired height. Hold in place with hairgrips (bobby pins) and hairspray.

PUMP UP THE VOLUME

For a cheap body-building hairspray, mix two cups of water with the juice of one orange in a saucepan. Bring slowly to the boil then cool and strain the mixture. Pour into a spray bottle and use it on wet hair to add volume.

SAY 'YES' TO SURVEYS

Save money on hair products by going online. Beauty suppliers often give away free samples of shampoo, conditioners and hair dyes in return for filling out surveys or joining a mailing list.

TANGLE-FREE TRESSES

Run out of detangler? Fabric softener can reduce hair static to prevent tangles. Make sure you read the label first though, to ensure that it doesn't contain bleach or colouring agents. Dilute with 12 parts water and apply a little to your hair after shampooing, then rinse it off immediately.

LESS IS MORE

Only spritz your hair three times with hairspray. Not only is this economical but too much spray can weigh down your hair and leave it looking flat.

MIGHTY MOUSSE

Make your own hair mousse by beating one egg white until it forms stiff peaks. Use your fingers to rub a tiny bit of whipped egg white into your hair and then style. This trick is used by hairdressers for catwalk shows as it gives amazing hold.

DO-IT-YOURSELF BLOW-DRY

To achieve a professional-looking blow-dry, apply a little mousse or styling lotion. Use a flat paddle brush or rounded brush while drying and finish with a spritz of serum for gloss and hairspray for hold.

HOMEMADE HAIR GEL

Making your own hair gel is an easy way to save money. Dissolve
½ teaspoon of gelatine in a cup of warm water, adding more gelatine
as needed to reach the desired consistency. Store in the refrigerator
between uses.

BRUSH EXTENDER

There's no need to throw out old hairbrushes and buy new ones.
Simply clean brushes by soaking them in a mild shampoo.

ZIG AND ZAG

If your roots are beginning to show why not put off your visit to the
salon a bit longer by experimenting with a new style? Try styling your
parting in a zigzag to hide your roots and make your hair look thicker.

FINE HAIR SOLUTION

Spend wisely and check the labels. Look out for products that contain
proteins (keratin and collagen), silicone polymers or polymeric
quaternium compounds. These are chemicals that stick to the hair
shaft and make your hair appear thicker.

SWAP SHOP

If you and your mates are suckers for new products, why not get
together to discuss which ones you want to try and then take turns to
buy the products? This way you can all give them a go and you'll split
the cost of experimenting with products that may not work for you.

GO THE DISTANCE

Ever wonder why professional blow-dries last longer than when you
style your hair at home? The secret's in the cool air. Heat from the
hairdryer opens the cuticles and allows a style to be formed, but it's
the cool air that sets the style. So when you're blow-drying, finish each
section with a blast of cooler air.

DIVIDE AND CONQUER
When drying hair, make like your hairstylist and divide it into several manageable sections, of 5–10 cm (2–4 in) thickness. That way you can focus on styling one section and clip the rest of the hair out of the way.

THE STRAIGHT STORY
The hairstylist's secret for blow-drying hair straight is all about angles. To get that super-sleek look, the airflow from the blow-dryer needs to be directed down the hair shaft, from the roots towards the ends.

CURL BOOSTING
Curl-boosting products can be expensive, so why not improvise? Simply rub a little of your usual conditioner between your hands then scrunch into your hair. It creates a more natural finish when dry than using mousses or gels.

DO-IT-YOURSELF UPDO
Don't pay someone to put your hair up – do it yourself. Pull your hair back as if you are gathering it in a ponytail at the base of your neck. Twist in an anticlockwise (counter-clockwise) motion, then keeping your hair taut, pull it up. Use one hand to hold the twist flat against your head. Tuck the 'tail' of the hair around your fingers and underneath, securing with hairgrips (bobby pins).

value hair treatments

PRICE MATCHING

Many salons will reduce the cost of your haircut if you tell them that you know you can get it cheaper across the street. Always ask if your salon will match a nearby competitor's price.

SAVE ON STYLISTS

If you go to a salon that offers different stylists at different prices, have your first cut and restyle with a senior stylist to ensure you get the shape and look just right then book follow-up trims with a junior stylist to save money.

BACK TO SCHOOL

For a big-salon cut without the big-salon price, ask if your salon has a training facility that you can visit, or enquire at a nearby hairdressing school. You'll get a discounted cut from a supervised trainee stylist.

DITCH THE DRYER

Leaving the salon with wet or roughly dried hair is always cheaper than letting the stylist dry and style it for you. The downside is that you don't get to see the finished look, but for long-hair trims and simple bobs it's a great way to save cash. Some salons will let you use their blow-dryers, too.

BRING ON THE BARBER'S

Are you a woman with a very straightforward cut? Then head to the local barber's shop. You'll pay a lot less than you would at a salon that caters solely for women, and a barber is usually just as experienced.

BECOME A HAIR MODEL

Willing to take risks with your hair? Then contact the top salons in your area and let them know that you're interested in becoming a hair model. You're more likely to bag a free cut if you have long hair that hasn't been chemically treated and you need to be open to a dramatic change of style and colour.

THINK A-HEAD

If you know your hair needs to be trimmed every six weeks it might be a wise idea to pre-book all your appointments in advance. A lot of stylists will reward your loyalty by knocking some money off your bill.

STRETCH IT OUT

Just because your stylist says you should come in every six weeks, that doesn't mean you have to. By lengthening the time between cuts to eight weeks you will shave two visits off of your yearly total.

STYLE FOR A SNIP

Plenty of high-end salons slash their prices during weekday afternoons when they're at their quietest. Don't be afraid to go inside and ask for details even if it's not advertised.

IN-BETWEEN FREEBIES

Many salons offer a free in-between-appointment trim for your fringe (bangs), as this is usually the first area to grow out. Take advantage of this when all you need is a tidy-up.

SAVE A BUNDLE

The more treatments you have from one salon, the cheaper the price will be for the individual treatments. Instead of making separate appointments for cut, colour and manicure, book all your services for the same day. You may get a chunk off the bill or they may throw in a blow-dry for free.

CHECK OUT COUPONS

Scour your local newspaper for salon vouchers. If you don't find any savings then go online. Start your search using the names of salons in your area and the word 'coupon'.

NEW ARRIVALS

Keep an eye out for new salons opening in your local area. They nearly always run special promotions to attract new customers. Spot one in your area and you could be rewarded with a half-price cut.

SAVE OR SPLURGE?

If you have your hair coloured professionally at a top salon, don't feel that you have to get it cut at the same time. If you've got a simple one-length style it might be worth getting it trimmed at a cheaper salon.

FACE UP TO IT

Achieve a rich highlighted effect by requesting colour highlights (or lowlights) only around your face. Partial highlights are cheaper than a whole or half head and will make a real difference as the hair next to your face is what people notice most. Alternatively ask for 'hidden' colour, where partial-head highlights are added to underneath sections so regrowth isn't obvious.

STAND THE TEST OF TIME

If you can't resist getting a professional blow-dry, make it go an extra day or two by asking the stylist to use rollers instead of just a rounded brush. Drying with rollers will give a longer-lasting bounce.

CUT THE COLOUR

High-maintenance colours – like light blonde or red – require frequent touch-ups that can be expensive. If you want great hair on a budget it's best to stay as close as possible to your natural colour and choose scattered highlights so that your roots are not obvious.

JOIN THE BRAIDY BUNCH

Can't afford to touch up dark roots? Plaiting (braiding) hair with regrowth is a favourite celebrity trick, and a great way to make a feature of the regrowth, as the contrast of colours can be striking. Any style that doesn't show the parting will hide regrowth, too, such as using hairbands or twisting the front section back to cover the crown.

STAGGER COLOUR

If you have a full head of highlights, save money by not getting a full colour each time your roots start to show. Use a three-visit cycle: on the first visit get the full head of highlights, then on the next two visits just get half a head.

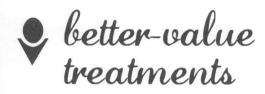

better-value treatments

CHIP AWAY THE COST

Chipping a recent manicure or pedicure is irritating. But don't worry – most nail salons offer a touch-up service that's cheaper than a full treatment. Go to your salon, taking the nail polish you used, and they'll make your nails look good as new in minutes.

FRIENDLY FREEBIES

Spas often have a 'take a friend for free' deal. Find yourself a partner in crime and you can grab great deals by splitting the cost. You may have to share a room, though, so make sure it's someone you get along well with!

LAST-MINUTE DEALS

Many hotels have a spa facility. They might not be as large as a dedicated spa, but if you just fancy lounging around in a pool and maybe having a facial, then you can save money by searching for a hotel with a spa on a last-minute travel website.

PRACTICE MAKES PERFECT

Beauty therapists learn their trade at beauty colleges. So if you fancy a cheap massage or beauty treatment, and you're willing to forego some of the trimmings, then find out whether your local college offers treatments by trainees.

MIDWEEK MONEY SAVING

People usually visit at the weekend, so spas nearly always have weekday spaces to fill. Ask if they offer discounted prices for midweek stays. You're bound to find a cheaper deal if you're flexible on which nights of the week you visit.

HOST A PAMPERING PARTY

Invite over a group of mates who all want a beauty treatment. If you tell a local home-visit beauty therapist that you will have 10 to 20 customers for them, you'll be able to negotiate a discounted rate. Aim for 20% off per person.

TREAT YOURSELF

Facials can be expensive, but there's a sneaky way to get more for your money. Beauty counters in department stores will often offer a free mini-facial if you buy at least two products from their range.

PHONE A FRIEND

Beauty therapists are always on the lookout for new clients, and will often show their appreciation with a free treatment if you refer a friend to them. Don't be afraid to ask.

LOYALTY CARD

Ask if your spa or salon offers rewards for loyalty. Many will give out cards on which you record your treatments and then after a certain number of visits you'll be rewarded with a free treatment.

BE IN THE KNOW

Always ask to be put on mailing lists for salons and cosmetic stores. You'll receive coupons and notices about upcoming specials and promotions, so you'll never miss a bargain.

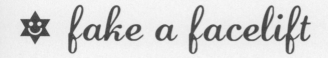 # fake a facelift

WORK OUT WORRY

To minimize frown lines, rub your temples and forehead with your knuckles. Start from the centre of your forehead and move out towards the temples. Massage for two minutes to ease the appearance of wrinkles. This also relieves headaches.

CREATE A YOUTHFUL GLOW

Apply cream pearl highlighter to your brow bone, the top of your cheeks and the inner corner of your eyes. This will lift your complexion, making you look younger in the process.

KEEP AN EYE ON AGEING

Having perfectly groomed eyebrows helps create the illusion of lifted lids. Plus, having more skin showing between your brow bone and eyelid opens up the entire eye area for a more fresh-faced look.

INVEST FOR SUCCESS

Skip the expensive Botox and invest in a skin-brightening face cream instead. These tighten your skin and leave your complexion looking radiant, knocking years off in the process.

BANISH BAGS

To fight discoloration and bags under the eyes, rub your face gently on either side of your nostrils. Gently rubbing here releases the toxins that can otherwise show up as blotches and bags under your eyes.

CLEVER COMBING

To make the skin on your face look instantly tighter and lifted, try this much-used celebrity favourite. Pull your hair back as tightly as is comfortable from your face and secure in place with hairgrips (bobby pins).

LIFT DROOPY EYES

Draw a line along your upper lashes with eyeliner, extending slightly further than the outer corner, and sloping upwards slightly. Line the bottom eyelid with a lighter shade to add to the lift effect.

YOUTHFUL PEEPERS

Cut out salty foods for at least three hours before bed. Salt triggers water retention, which can cause puffy eyes the next morning.

WIDE-AWAKE CLUB

Place three fingers under your eye and very gently pull down without closing your eyes. Hold for ten seconds and release. This will get the blood flowing to the skin under your eyes, which will help reduce puffiness.

FORGET TO FROWN

Stop worrying about laughter lines and smile! Over the years our faces lose fat and our brows lower, which makes your face look serious or cross in repose. But when you smile, your face lifts and your cheeks become rounder and more youthful. Smiling is the most natural facelift you can get.

LOSE YOUR LINES

To tone your cheeks and lessen the appearance of lateral lines, inhale and hold the air in your mouth with your cheeks puffed out like a trumpet player. Hold for as long as you can before slowly exhaling through your nostrils. Repeat five times. This is also a good stress-buster.

NATURAL NIP AND TUCK

Hold the underside of your chin with an open palm. Tilt your head back until you feel your throat skin stretching. Intensify the stretch by bringing your lower lip up over the upper one. Hold for 20 seconds and repeat ten times every day.

fake a nose job

CREATE WIDER APPEAL

Apply a broad strip of highlighter or pale powder down the centre of your nose and blend well using a lighter foundation to enlarge a nose that's too thin.

THE PINOCCHIO EFFECT

Apply highlighter or pale powder over and under the tip of your nose. By drawing attention to the tip of your nose you will make it seem more prominent.

PERFECT POWDER

Highlights and shine tend to draw attention to features. However, matt powder applied to the nose will make it appear smaller.

AVOID POINTING IT OUT

A centre parting is like an arrow pointing directly to your nose, so opt for a side parting instead. If your nose bends slightly to one side, part your hair on the opposite side to help balance it.

HAVE A RESTYLE

Talk to your hairstylist about styles that will best suit your face. Bear in mind that short, straight styles tend to emphasize the nose so opt for long, wavy locks instead.

SLIM YOUR SNOUT

To create the illusion of a narrower nose, apply a matt bronzer down the sides of your nose. Then apply a thin stripe of pale powder highlighter down the bridge of your nose. Make sure to blend well to avoid a streaky finish.

DON'T BE BLUNT

Thick, blunt fringes (bangs) can look like a pelmet highlighting a larger nose. Softer, side-sweeping fringes are more flattering.

GET SHORTY

To make a long nose seem shorter, blend a slightly darker foundation under your nose and up over the tip. Extend your blush application to just below the apples of your cheeks. This will make your cheeks appear to end lower down your face, putting things in proportion.

MIND THE BUMP

To hide a crooked nose, apply bronzer down the bridge of your nose stopping where the tip begins to protrude. Be sure to blend it well. A straight line of highlighter down the centre will also help make it look straighter.

DISTRACTION TECHNIQUES

If you dislike your nose, choose flamboyant, statement earrings to help distract attention away from the centre of the face. Go for studs, however, as very dangly earrings can accentuate a longer nose.

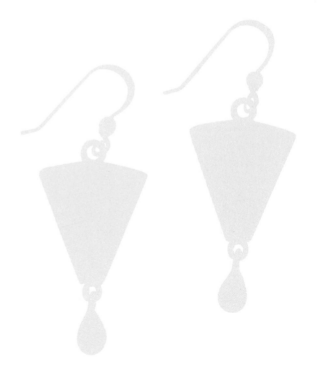

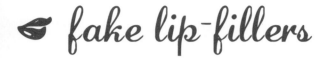 # fake lip-fillers

GLOSS OVER WEAKER POINTS

Make narrow lips appear fuller by applying a dab of gloss or a paler shade of lipstick in the centre of your lips to create the illusion of plumpness.

PENCIL IN YOUR POUT

Trace just outside your upper lip line using a slightly blunt lipliner. Fill in the new lip area with the pencil using very light pressure, so the outline still looks slightly darker. Then paint over the whole area with gloss.

PEARLY SMILE

Choose lipsticks with a pearlized, shimmery finish. Shine reflects light, which will make your lips look instantly plumper.

TAKE A LIGHTER APPROACH

If you have a small mouth, avoid dark lipsticks or glosses as they can make your lips look smaller. Instead, choose a lighter shade to give the illusion of fullness.

CAST A SHADOW

Dot a tiny amount of soft-brown eyeliner under your lower lip line. This creates the illusion that your full lips are creating a shadow. But remember a little goes a long way – use too much and you risk looking like you're growing a beard!

CLEVER CUPID

For a fuller-looking top lip, apply a highlighter or pale pink lip pencil to your Cupid's bow (the 'm' shape right above your upper lip).

fake a boob job

DRESS TO IMPRESS

A pretty fitted top with a narrow V-neck will accentuate a small bust. Ruffles, lace, breast pockets and wide collars will also give the illusion of larger breasts. But stay away from tops that are too big or flowing, or those with deep V-necks if you have a very small bust.

KEEP THEM CROSSED

Buy a multiway bra and position the straps so they cross over at the back. This will pull up your breasts and make them look larger.

ENHANCE YOUR ASSETS

Padded and push-up bras obviously enhance your bust and most men will never notice the effect as all breasts look different without a bra. Don't be tempted to go for ridiculous amounts of padding, though, or you do risk disappointing your partner!

ENHANCING EXERCISE

To enlarge the pectoral muscles under the breast tissue, put your hands in front of your chest in a praying position. Lift your elbows up and out and push your hands together really hard for a count of 20. Repeat ten times daily.

CLEVER CAMOUFLAGE

To make your breasts appear fuller and rounder, use a large brush to apply bronzer in back and forth strokes over the curve at the top of your breast. Then, using a thinner brush, apply a paler powder to the centre of your cleavage.

MAXIMIZING MASSAGE

For plumper breasts on a night out, massage all around them with a bust cream to get the blood circulation flowing.

BE UPFRONT

If you're wearing a top you want to enhance your cleavage in, choose a bra that fastens at the front. This allows you to push your breasts up and closer together more easily.

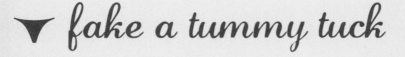

fake a tummy tuck

BLOAT-BUSTING EPSOM

Epsom salts are commonly used by naturopaths and osteopaths to ease stress and flush out toxins, but they are also one of the cheapest, simplest ways to reduce tummy swelling. Buy at the pharmacy and dissolve a large handful in hot bath water.

BE A CLING-ON

For an instantly smoother silhouette, wrap cling film (plastic wrap) around your tummy and thighs before going for a jog or working out. The sweating effect this triggers will temporarily reduce water retention and banish bloating – a fabulous quick fix if you need to squeeze into that little black dress.

SHAPING SQUATS

Squat up and down, touching the ground with your fingers, as fast as you can for a minute. This causes an oxygen deficit within your body, which forces your body to burn fat for energy. And, because it's close to the heart, fat from your middle will be the first to go.

MAGIC KNICKERS

Gripper knickers have revolutionized the underwear industry. Never before has underwear had the power to slim and smooth your belly. If you need to hide a muffin-top then go for entire body shapers.

PERFECT POSTURE

Straighten up and pull your stomach muscles in towards your spine – your figure will instantly look sleeker. Plus, when your posture is good you're automatically engaging and toning your stomach muscles.

JUMP FOR FLAT-STOMACH JOY

Invest in a mini-home trampoline. Bouncing on one in short five-minute bursts with ten-minute breaks in between helps tone weak tummy muscles.

DRINK YOURSELF THIN

Being dehydrated causes the body to store excess water, which can lead you to carry up to 1.75 kg (4 lb) of excess weight around your middle. Try to drink six to eight glasses of water daily to prevent this.

 # *sun-protection savings*

SENSITIVE SUNBLOCK

Don't pay extra for a specialized sunscreen if you have sensitive skin. Just shop around for one with a very simple ingredients list, containing only the physical ingredients zinc oxide or titanium dioxide. Unlike chemical sunscreen agents, which absorb UV rays, it's rare to have an allergy to physical sunscreens.

AVOID BREAKOUTS

You don't need an expensive oil-free sunscreen to prevent breakouts; just look for one that is water or gel based. It's a bonus if you can find one that is fragrance-free.

DON'T OVERSTOCK

Sunscreen doesn't last very long – heat and bacteria damage it over time. Don't be tempted to bulk-buy when you see special offers unless you know you're going to use it. Discard any that is past the expiration date.

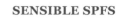

SENSIBLE SPFS

You should always wear at least SPF 15 to protect your skin. So anything with an SPF lower than this is a waste of money when it comes to preventing skin damage or premature ageing.

TWO FOR ONE

Make sure you buy a 'broad spectrum' sunscreen that protects you from both UVA and UVB rays. You really need to protect against both so there's no point buying a bottle that only shields your skin from one.

INSPECT THE INGREDIENTS

Sunscreen doesn't need to be expensive to be effective. As long as zinc oxide, titanium dioxide or avobenzone are listed as ingredients you should be in safe hands.

MULTIPURPOSE MOISTURIZER

If you prefer the shade and don't plan to expose a lot of skin to the sun you can swap sunscreen for an inexpensive facial moisturizer with an SPF. Apply to your face, neck and hands every day.

BUY BEFORE YOU FLY

Stores in popular tourist destinations tend to bump up the price of sunscreen as they know they will have a captive audience. Buy before you fly to save a little cash.

EARLY APPLICATION

Why spend money on a product that isn't going to work because you don't use it properly? Follow the golden sunscreen rule, which means applying half an hour before you go out in the sun for it to be effective.

BE GENEROUS

Don't be stingy when applying sunscreen. For this reason, it's better to buy a cheap (but effective) sunscreen, as you won't need to worry about how much you slather on.

HERE'S THE RUB...

Even waterproof sunscreen can't withstand towel-drying so always reapply sunscreen after drying yourself, or alternatively let yourself air-dry. Either way, treatment for sunburn will cost far more than using enough sunscreen.

LIFESAVER

If sunscreen starts to smell funny or separates, you should get rid of it because it won't work properly. However, you can prolong the life of your sunscreen by storing it in the refrigerator and keeping it in the shade while you're on the beach.

AFTER SUN

It's important to moisturize your skin after sun exposure, but don't feel the need to buy expensive after-sun products – normal moisturizers or body lotions will work just as well. Add a dollop of aloe vera gel to soothe sore skin.

IN THE SWIM

If you are going swimming make sure your sunscreen won't wash off the second you hit the water. Generally, a sunscreen that is 'water repellent' will withstand two 20-minute swims. While one that is 'waterproof' will withstand four 20-minute dips. Check the details on the bottle you buy.

PRICELESS PRODUCT

The only skincare product that can slow the ageing process, reduce scarring and acne, all but eliminate wrinkles and even prevent cancer, is sunscreen. When you consider the amount of money spent on plastic surgery and cosmetics, it's a wonder why anyone wouldn't use sunscreen daily. It's the most important and cost-effective part of your skincare routine.

✔ supplements: the hits

COD LIVER OIL

Any omega-3-loaded fish oil will help maintain and build supple skin, lustrous hair and stronger nails. It can also help improve the texture of bumpy skin on the tops of your arms.

PROTEIN POWER

Studies have shown biotin supplements can strengthen dry, brittle nails, making them a worthwhile beauty investment.

LOTTA BOTTLE

Research by Swedish scientists has found that yogurt and yogurt-type digestion-improving drinks – the type that contain friendly bacteria known as probiotics – do work and also boost the immune system. A bottle a day should leave you less bloated and looking and feeling more energized.

MAGNESIUM OK

Women are often low in this mineral, so a supplement can help ease PMS symptoms and reduce monthly skin breakouts.

SUPER SILICA

This natural mineral is necessary for healthy hair, skin and nails. Taking a supplement will improve hair thickness, skin tone and nail strength. It is also widely promoted for the prevention of osteoporosis.

ZINC FOR ZITS

Acne is often linked to zinc deficiency. A dose of 30 mg per day can improve your skin. But get the right type – zinc picolinate is the easiest to absorb, so you may be wasting your money if you buy other forms that often pass straight through the body.

EVENING, PRIMROSE

One of the most concentrated sources of gama linoleic acid (GLA)
– an essential fatty acid – is evening primrose oil. GLAs have anti-
inflammatory properties and play an important role in maintaining
hormone balance and healthy skin – they can help treat dry or acne-
prone skin and even eczema. Evening primrose is also said to improve
the condition of nails, scalp and hair, so it may be worth trying.

✗ when to save:
the misses

EAT IT UP

You only need a tiny amount of the mineral selenium and this can
easily be obtained from meat, nuts, bread, fish or eggs. Taking a
supplement will increase the chances of absorbing too much, which
can actually lead to weaker skin, hair and nails.

C CLEARLY

There are no scientific studies that show that taking vitamin C as a
supplement has any effect on improving skin.

COLLAGEN CAPSULES

As the body gets older it stops producing collagen but taking
supplements won't help you regain a youthful appearance. According
to the British Skin Foundation, there's no evidence to support the
idea that oral collagen supplements prevent wrinkles or improve the
condition of your skin.

B COMPLEX

While B vitamins are vital for healthy skin, hair and nails, you're
better off getting your daily dose from food, as overdosing is easy
and can lead to nasty side effects such as chest pain, fatigue, stomach
upset, depression or numbness.

AIN'T NO SUNSHINE

Tan-optimizing pills aren't a great idea as they can provide a false sense of security, meaning you end up spending longer in the sun and causing damage to your skin. A tan is a sign of damaged skin and there's no such thing as a safe tan. You're better off spending your pennies on a fake tan with a high SPF built in.

KEEP IT REAL

There's no proof that taking synthesized supplements of single antioxidants will keep skin young. It's thought that antioxidants probably only work as part of a food as they may need other components of the food to be effective.

NOT A-LIST

Vitamin A (retinol) helps keep skin healthy. But a woman needs just 0.6 mg a day, according to the UK's Food Standards Agency, which means you can get all you need from foods such as cheese, eggs, oily fish, milk and yogurt. More than 1.5 mg per day may actually make your bones more brittle and prone to fracture as you age.

E-ASY DOES IT

Vitamin E helps protect cell membranes by acting as an antioxidant. While it may be moisturizing, taking a supplement can't actually fight ageing or prevent wrinkles.

WATER WORKS

So-called 'beauty waters' can be a waste of money because often the vitamins or herbs they contain are in such tiny amounts they're unlikely to have any effect. Also they often contain sugar or artificial sweeteners, in which case you'd be better off having a glass of ordinary water from the tap (faucet).

WRINKLE RIP-OFF?

Thinking of buying an expensive anti-ageing vitamin formula? Bear in mind there's no proven research that taking a pill each day will improve wrinkles or stop them from forming.

how to haggle

BE COURAGEOUS

Don't be afraid to haggle, even in a department store or beauty salon chain. The worst that can happen is they say 'no'. And if you're successful you'll leave glowing with the knowledge that you just paid less than everyone else for your haircut/massage/lipstick.

A RIGHT CHARMER

But do remember that aggressive or forceful haggling is a mistake as it annoys the person you're dealing with. You'll get further if you're polite, charming and treat the situation with humour.

AVOID AN AUDIENCE

Anyone in a position to decide the price of something is usually aware that if other people are around there's a risk that they too will want a discount. So be discreet and haggle quietly to allow the person in charge to be more flexible.

LOOK FOR LAZY LABELLING

Don't just take the first product you see to the cashdesk. It's worth rifling through the shelf in search of the one item that's been mispriced or carries an earlier price. You can then demand the store honour the tag!

CREATE A PRICE WAR

Shop around before you haggle. If you know you can get an item or service cheaper elsewhere then tell the sales assistant/beauty therapist and they may well offer you a deal to secure your custom. The more stores you play against each other, the better your chance of bagging a bargain.

SHOW AN INTEREST

When buying a beauty product or receiving a beauty treatment, ask about the other products and services they offer. Ask lots of questions and show a real interest and you may be offered a free sample or trial.

IT'S A GIFT!

When purchasing a beauty product or perfume tell the salesperson that it's a gift. They may throw some free samples into your bag as an extra treat or at the very least offer you prettier packaging!

INTERNET INVESTIGATION

Many retailers operate online and have stores on the web, with the online price invariably being cheaper than in their individual outlets. If you print out their online price and ask them to match it in-store you can save on the delivery fee.

BUILD A RELATIONSHIP

If you always buy your beauty products from the same salesperson or your treatments from the same beauty therapist, you'll soon build up a friendly relationship with them. And from time to time they may reward your loyalty with freebies or a 10% discount.

DEAL WITH DECISION MAKERS

If a salesperson doesn't have the power to give you a discount, then find out who does. In chain stores, that's typically a manager or supervisor. The same holds true when you're negotiating fees for beauty treatments.

SPOT IMPERFECTIONS

Always point out any flaws in the product, for example if the packaging is damaged, and ask for a discount.

TIMING IS EVERYTHING

Don't try to haggle on a busy Saturday afternoon. There's no reason for a sales assistant to offer a reduction when they have plenty of other customers willing to pay full price. Weekdays and early mornings are the best time to ask for money off.

SERVICE SWAP

If you're willing to design and hand out flyers for your hairstylist or beauty therapist, they may offer you a free cut or at least a discounted rate in return for your marketing services.

SUPERSIZE SALE BARGAINS

If the price is already reduced, such as during a sale, there is often greater flexibility. Sales are designed to clear room for new stock, so managers are often willing to accept lower than the marked sale price. A bit of cheeky haggling might see you being offered extra discounts.

SLEUTH FOR PRE-SALES

Stores rarely put all their stock on sale at once, but if some products are discounted it is always worth asking if the one you want is due to be in the sale too. Chances are the retailer may be able to sell it at sale price if you ask nicely.

BLAME YOUR OTHER HALF

When deciding whether to buy an extra product or treatment a good line to try is 'I would love to buy this, but my husband/boyfriend will go mad if I pay this amount'. A sales assistant who empathizes could well knock a little money off.

STAY IN TOUCH

Always ask to go on the mailing list at stores and salons. This will keep you informed of any special-offer evenings or discreet deals for valued customers.

DON'T BE AFRAID OF SILENCE

When haggling it pays to pause. Let the sales assistant fill the gaps in the conversation with better offers.

ASK FOR A CASH DISCOUNT

Offer to pay in cash. You may just save yourself another 10%. Many credit card companies charge stores a fee for every transaction they carry out, therefore some stores offer a discount on goods for a cash sale. This applies particularly to the smaller independent stores.

THREATEN TO QUIT

If you have a membership at a gym, or a longstanding relationship with a beauty salon, tell them that you dearly want to stay but you've seen too many better deals elsewhere, then see what they offer.

BULK-BUY BARGAINING

Discounts are more often available if you're buying a lot of items in one go. So if you're going to buy a few products from the same range, or are planning to stock up on your favourite, it's always worth asking if you've earned a discount. Why not get together a few friends who are after the same thing?

PICK YOUR BATTLES

You're much more likely to be able to haggle for bargains in independent stores or salons than you are in major chains.
Any store or salon where you can speak directly to the owner is a better bet, as they will have the authority to negotiate.

final freebies

SAVVY SAMPLES

When buying make-up or beauty products always insist on having a sample first. Your skin, hair and colouring are unique so you have the right to ensure that products work for you before you invest in them.

FRIENDLY FREEBIES

It always pays to have friends in the beauty industry. They'll often be sent more free samples than they can use, so if they're feeling generous they may let you take some off their hands.

VALUABLE VOUCHERS

There are many websites that offer voucher codes that you can use in stores or online. Just enter the name of the brand you are looking for and 'money off' into a search engine and you could find vouchers for free delivery or up to 20% off.

CARRY AN EMPTY

Want to try a beauty product but they don't have a ready-to-go sample? Whip out your own container and they'll have no excuse for saying no!

PERFECT PROMOTIONS

If you can, wait until your favourite brand is running a promotion in department stores or pharmacies. You'll often get a free bag of goodies with your purchase.

WATCH OUT FOR ADS

The newer the product, the greater the marketing budget, which means you're more likely to get your hands on a free sample.

READ ALL ABOUT IT

Keep an eye out in newspapers and magazines for reader's trial panels. You'll be sent free samples of beauty products for you to try and review.

MASTER MARKET RESEARCH

Sign up to online market research companies or take part in street surveys. The researchers will often offer free samples to people who are willing to give them feedback on new products.

POCKET SAMPLES

Whether you are in the hair salon or dentist's waiting room, don't pass up the opportunity to flick through glossy magazines. They often have mini hair and skin samples you can pocket. After all, why let them go to waste?

BE PAID TO SHOP

Get a store card for the introductory offer, then pay the bill asap and cut up the card. Alternatively, use cash-back credit cards and pay off the monthly balance in full.

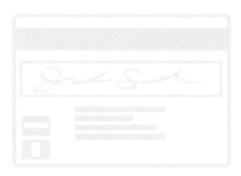

index